What people are say

"When I came to Edu _____ *orso and no function in my* _____ *had a return of my back and abdomen muscles and can walk three hundred fifty steps in the LiteGait® machine and do a hundred squats every time I visit Edward's office. Working with him has been a miracle in my life."*

– Karen David

"This book is a roadmap to lifelong health based upon a natural, holistic, and effective approach. Each chapter is packed with one breakthrough insight after another."

– Dr. Woody Beck, D.C., Q.N.

"Medical doctors had all but given up on me, and then I met Dr. Edward Chauvin. My left side was paralyzed, and after years of traditional treatments, I had not restored any neurological functions. With Edward's help and Quantum Neurology® techniques, I believe I will be back to a hundred percent very soon."

– Roger Sims

"I truly respect Dr. Chauvin, and I know that this book will be of service to those who allow themselves to be served by the years of applied knowledge and care to which Dr. Chauvin has dedicated himself."

– Dr. James D. Sheen, D.C.

"Thanks to Quantum Neurology® and Dr. Chauvin, I am no longer borderline leukemia, my leukemia risk is gone, MSA symptoms have been minimized, and people keep asking me if I had a face lift. It's from getting neurological function back in my face, not from any surgery."

– Dr. Sue Lein

"Dr. Chauvin's ability to find and repair problems in the human body is absolutely incredible. He is my doctor and I truly believe that he is one of the best doctors in the world."

– Dr. Chris Cormier, D.C., Author of The Hidden Diagnosis& Health Product Formulator

I'm Worried Sick About My Health

How to Get and Stay Healthy Without Spending a Fortune

I'm Worried Sick About My Health

How to Get and Stay Healthy Without Spending a Fortune

Edward R. Chauvin, D.C.

ISBN: 978-1479342105

Book Cover Design by Cathi Stevenson
www.BookCoverExpress.com

Interior Design by Rudy Milanovich
rudy@WizardVision.net

Book Edited by Maura Leon
www.MauraLeon.com

"The doctor of the future will give no medicine, but will interest his patients in the care of the human frame, in diet, and in the cause and prevention of disease."

—Thomas Edison, Inventor

Dedication

I would like to first thank my Lord and Savior, Jesus Christ. While growing up, I had a school counselor who told me I wasn't smart enough to go to college and I should think about joining the military. But the Spirit of God within me said, "I can do all things through Christ who strengthens me," (Philippians 4:13) so I prayed, I studied hard, and I graduated with honor from chiropractic college. Please don't listen to the negative voices of others, or the negative voices that are sometimes in your head, saying things like, *I'm not good enough; I'm not smart enough; I'm not talented enough; I'm not tall enough; I'm not short enough; I'm not skinny enough or not fat enough.* All you need to do is "seek first the kingdom of God and His righteousness, and all these things shall be added unto you" as well. (Matthew 6:33) When I think of my life and its importance, nothing compares to my belief that He is for us, and "if God is for us, who can be against us?" (Romans 8:31)

I have three wonderful children who have blessed my life with so much happiness and fulfillment: my oldest son, Benjamin Edward Chauvin; my second son, Patrick Jerry Chauvin; and my daughter, Jasmine Nicole Chauvin. I dedicate this book to them, that they might read it and see that they should follow me, as I follow Christ, and never give up on the goals that God has placed in their hearts, to choose health and good things, daily, and never be worried that God's word will not stand in all the resistance that may come against them from life. Children, remember that the word of God says, "many are the afflictions of the righteous, but the Lord delivers him out of them all." (Psalms 34:19). The choices are yours to be healthy and happy. It's called the good fight of faith, but "faith without works is dead," (James 2:20) so work at it every day. Remember how much your father loves you. You are smart; you are strong; you are healthy; you are able to accomplish anything, with God, if you work hard at it and never give up. Speak positively, think positively, and be great. I see greatness in each one of you. You "can do all things through Christ who strengthens" you.

(Philippians 4:13)

Contents

Acknowledgements

Thanks to my mother for all the prayers she has said, and continues to say, for me.

Thanks to Edna Greene, or "Mutsy," as we used to call her, who showed me all the love that a person as white as I am would need to feel from a black woman. I miss her terribly.

Thanks to my dad, who showed me an extremely good work ethic and how to be my best at all times.

Thanks to my big brother, Jay Chauvin, who put up the five thousand dollars I needed to be transported by helicopter to Shreveport from Lafayette when the aneurism ruptured. He did it without blinking. He is one of my heroes.

Thanks to Jesse Wilder, who showed me that honest, hard work always pays off.

Thanks to R.L. Savoy, who was my chiropractic father and the one who got me interested in practicing chiropractic.

Thanks to Dr. Julian Bailes, who was my roommate in college and who saved my life, in 2007, by performing neurosurgery on a class five aneurysm rupture. I thank God for him every day.

Thanks to Dr. George Gonzalez, who discovered and taught me Quantum Neurology® and was also instrumental in the recovery of all my neurological functions after my surgery in 2007. He is the reason that this book is being written, as he helped me to see not only that I could do it but that it would be good for my lifetime and beyond.

Thanks to Dr. Chris Cormier for pushing me to write my story.

Thanks to Dr. James Sheen, a Quantum Neurologist™ from Nebraska, whom we like to call "Einstein" because his mind is so sharp with the new concepts and scores of information that he remembers, in detail, about how to apply those concepts to help people get well. I'm glad to say that he is my friend.

Thanks to Dr. David Kats from Kats Management, who showed me how to run a chiropractic office using moral and ethical methods.

Thanks to Dr. Walter Vern Pierce, who was the best chiropractic adjuster and the most outspoken man I've ever known. His ideas of adjusting the spine are still the best that I know of.

Thanks to Keith Leon, my book mentor. This book would not have happened if it was not for Keith. He promised he would "make the writing process easy" and he made good on that promise. I'm grateful that God brought us together so this book can find its way to those who are ready to receive its message.

Thanks to Maura Leon for the beautiful job she has done editing this book and helping me get my voice to the people who need to hear it in this way.

Thanks to Rudy Milanovich for the beautiful book layout.

Thanks to Cathi Stevenson for doing such a great job on the book cover. It far exceeded my expectations.

And thanks to all of my patients, who have taught me so much about health and about myself. God has truly blessed me with the best people in the whole world as my patients!

Foreword

I like to say that God has a picture of Edward Chauvin in his wallet. By the time you finish reading his book, I think you will agree. I assure you that Edward is very human, with ups and downs in life, just as we all have, but there is something about a person who did not break one bone after being hit by a car and having his knees pinned to the wall by the car's bumper. He also survived been impaled by a steel rod that went from his groin into his upper chest without piercing an organ. And in this book you will hear Edward's account of surviving a grade five brain aneurysm with zero neurological deficits, and how he went back to work, practicing full time, the next month!

As the developer of a nervous system rehabilitation system called Quantum Neurology®, I have seen lots of miraculous healing events through my work. I developed this system through the rehabilitation and full recovery of my wife's moderate spinal cord injury. Her healing, and her ability to then have our daughter, is my personal miracle. I have taught this work to many doctors around the world and I am blessed to call Dr. Edward Chauvin my student and friend.

Edward's ability to live through just one of these events is impressive, but to thrive after three of them is no doubt a miracle. It should not surprise you that Edward is strong in prayer and faith. I have always been on a spiritual path, but until I had met Edward I had no idea what it meant to be focused in prayer.

The first time I visited Edward in his home town of Abbeville, Louisiana, I was doing FDA submitted research on light therapy. He is one of the highest trained practitioners of Quantum Neurology® and I was excited to see how he had integrated my work into his practice and why he was so successful at activating healing in his patients. It did not take very long before I recognized that he brings more to the table than the learned skills of nervous system rehabilitation. As he works with his patients, Edward is in a constant conversation of gratitude with God. Two patients told me that they became cancer free after he had prayed for them. Several would cry while sharing their story of suffering, and then healing, through his care. In his office, I have personally witnessed paralyzed patients rehabilitating and walking out of their wheelchairs. Other patients return to report that their diseases, verified by blood work, are no longer present.

Albert Einstein said, "There are two ways to live: you can live as if nothing is a miracle; you can live as if everything is a miracle." Edward lives his life as if everything is a miracle. He works hard, he plays hard, and he loves hard. If you were to ask Edward why he survived these accidents and his aneurysm, he would give glory to God. If you ask me, I have no doubt that God has bigger and better things planned for Edward…and this book is just the beginning.

With love, kindness, and gratitude,
Dr. George Gonzalez, D.C., QN, Chiropractor, Quantum Neurologist™ Founder of Quantum Neurology® Nervous System Rehabilitation, Author of the Holographic Healing™ series

Introduction

I've been a practicing chiropractor for over thirty years now and I've seen so many cases where God has used me in people's lives to influence and help. I have kept a folder with all of the incredible results that people have experienced after Quantum Neurology® and I thought to myself, *someday I will use these stories to write a book*. Well, I only procrastinated for twenty years…yes, for twenty years I have wanted to do this.

On one very special day, Dr. George Gonzalez looked at me and said, "Edward, you have to write your story. You have to tell people about what you're doing in your office and how God has worked with you, and through you, to create miracles."

At first I thought: *well, I've got a packet of information and I've got the title of my book already.* I've noticed, in my years as a chiropractor, that so many people are worried sick about their health but they're doing nothing about it. I thought this would be the best time to write the book, as Quantum Neurology® is just being birthed right now and people all over the world are finding out about it. I realized that this is the time that people need to know there is a natural way to get rid of the nerve interference in their life and to be healthy using diet, exercise, proper rest, a positive mental attitude, and freedom from nerve interference.

Next, my good friend and colleague, Dr. Chris Cormier, said, "You've got to write your book."

"Oh, come on, Chris, I'm not a writer. I read for information, not for fun. I don't do that stuff."

"Ed, just write your story. It's the best story I've ever heard and I've heard a lot of them. And you can tell it so well. Just write it.

"I have a book mentor I work with named Keith Leon. He's known as 'The Book Guy' and he helped me get my book edited, published, and out to the masses in record time. He'll work with you and walk you all the way through the process."

I contacted Keith and started working with him. He really did make the whole process easy and fun.

There are three main reasons why I wanted to write this book:

First, I've always wanted to hand a copy to my children so they read it and say, "My dad wrote this book!"

Second, I want my patients to read this book because I don't always have time to share my inspiring story with them in as much detail as this book has allowed. My hope is that my patients will share this book with people they know and care about so those folks will go see a Quantum Neurologist™ and get a natural approach to health, instead of going to a crisis care doctor. Seeing a crisis care doctor is not a bad thing, but if you've waited until that point then you are already in a world of hurt before you get to the Quantum Neurologist™. Why not start setting yourself up for health *before* you're in pain? Prevention is more effective than trying to reverse an already pain-filled diagnosis. I believe this book is an introduction that may lead someone to making this type of healthy choice, and this pleases me greatly.

And finally, I'd love it if this book led someone to God's word and caused them to put God first in their life and to realize that good health is an obtainable goal.

Chapter 1

My Chiropractic Miracle

When I was in high school I played football, and I played both offense and defense. In my junior year, I injured my back and went to my family physician. He told me I just had some muscle spasms and I should take the medicine he prescribed and the pain would go away in a few days.

Well, it didn't go away. I was in constant pain. My football coach looked at me and said, "Oh, you're just faking it. Get out there and play." I was in so much physical pain I could barely move.

After I had played through the pain as much as I could, my head coach said to me, "Edward, I have quite a few guys on the team who are seeing a chiropractor; perhaps you should see him to."

"What's a chiropractor?" I asked.

"Why don't you talk to Bobby about that. All I know is, Bobby goes and it helps him."

I talked to Bobby and what he shared encouraged me to make an appointment with the chiropractor he was seeing. His name was Dr. R. L. Savoy and he was located in Church Point, Louisiana. This was back in 1973 and chiropractors were not licensed in the state of Louisiana. As a matter of fact, Louisiana was the last state in the United States to license chiropractors. So when I got to this guy's office it was like no doctor's office I had ever seen before. It was dark in there and it was kind of spooky and scary. I was like, *wow, I don't even know if I want to go into this place*, but I was brave and I went in anyway.

Dr. Savoy met me and proceeded to take an X-ray of my lower back. He showed me the X-ray and said, "You see this bone right here. It's out of place. Can you see that?"

"Well, I don't know how to read X-rays doc, but it does look a little crooked to me."

The doctor told me he was going to put the bone back into place and I agreed that it was okay for him to do so. He put me on this chiropractic knee chest table (which I would not use today, but it served its purpose at the time). He looked at me and told me to relax. When he adjusted my spine, I thought to myself: *Oh my God, he just broke my back!* I was feeling energy move all throughout my body. I thought I was done for, but when I stood up, my back felt so much better and I said, "Wow, this feels great!"

I was able to play football for the rest of my junior and senior years of high school. I made several trips back to him, over the next few years, to get adjusted. I was really blown away by what he was doing and how effective his treatments were.

I moved on to college at Louisiana State University. I was trying to decide what I wanted to do there. I had grown up around horses, dogs, and other animals and at one time I thought I might want to become a veterinarian. After thinking about this for a while, I became clear that being a veterinarian was not what I wanted to do. But what was I going to study?

As I continued my inquiry, I remembered back to when I had played football and what this great chiropractor had done for me. I thought to myself: *Yes, that's what I want to do. I want to be a chiropractor.* Dr. Savoy had helped me so much when I needed it. The memories of how he had helped me made it clear that I wanted to help other people who were in pain just like I was. I wanted to be of service to others and help them in their time of need.

I called Dr. Savoy and told him that I would like to go to a chiropractic college and become a chiropractor. "It's funny that you would say that," he replied, "because I've already sent your name in to Palmer Chiropractic College, where I went to school, and told them that I felt you were a potential student."

My grades were pretty good at LSU, but they weren't the highest. I wasn't sure if they were high enough for me to be able to get into this college, but I applied anyway. Dr. Savoy was kind enough to send a letter of recommendation and I was accepted.

My mother was okay with my decision, saying, "Well, if that's really what you want to do. You know we don't really know much about chiropractors. You're the only one in the family who's ever been to one."

My father had a different reaction entirely: "Oh no, you cannot go. You cannot do this."

"Dad, this is what I want to do and I'm doing it."

"Well, I'm not helping you. You're going to have to do it on your own."

"I didn't ask for your help, Dad. I can do this myself."

The next day, I had my car packed and I was ready to go to Davenport, Iowa, which was a long way from Louisiana. When I arrived at the school, I was very disappointed. I was used to the grandness of LSU and all its buildings and stadiums. LSU was beautiful and spacious. Now I found myself at this small professional college and I thought to myself: *Oh no, this is the wrong place.*

I had a lot of judgment on its appearance when I first arrived, but I received a great education at Palmer. They focused purely on the study of chiropractic. There were no sports programs, no distractions. It was a wonderful time in my life and I learned so many great life lessons at that school. I graduated cum laude in my class with honors and I have been a chiropractor ever since.

My Personal Transformation

As I stated before, I had decided to become a chiropractor when I was at Louisiana State University back in 1975. My college roommate, Julian Bailes, had decided he would head off to medical school and went on to become a world-renowned neurosurgeon. On April 1, 2007, we had not spoken in at least eleven years because we were so involved with our studies at school, but everything was about to change forever.

I was working out with weights at my favorite health club. I recall that it was a heavy lifting day of my routine. As a matter of fact, on that day I benched four hundred pounds, ten times, which was a personal record of mine. I remember saying to myself, *man you are strong*, because this was the strongest I had ever been. I had never lifted that much weight. As I continued to lift weights, I started to feel nauseated. I entered the steam room, which I frequented regularly. While I was in the steam room, the nausea continued and my head began to ache.

My daughter was waiting for me outside of the health club, as she normally did, because we always went home from the club together. I thought to myself: *I'd better just stay here on the bench for a few minutes and gather my composure before I go off to meet my daughter.* After taking some time, I felt a little bit better so I went to the locker room to get dressed. I met my daughter, got into the car, and drove home. I don't, however, remember arriving at home.

The last thing I remember is getting to Maurice, Louisiana, which is about twelve miles from Abbeville, the town that I live in. My daughter looked at me and said, "Dad, you're sleeping."

I said, "No, Baby, I'm just resting my eyes right now."

I drove forward, out of an intersection, and that is the last thing I remember until I woke up in the hospital.

I had previously told my family that if I ever had a head injury, to make sure they called Julian Bailes because he was a great guy, I trusted him, and he was a great neurosurgeon. At that time, he was living in West Virginia and was head of the West Virginia School of Medicine.

My family attempted to contact Julian, thinking that he was in West Virginia, but Julian just happened to be in his hometown of Natchitoches, Louisiana, visiting his mother in the nursing home, when my family reached him. He instructed them to get me on the plane from Lafayette to Shreveport, where he would be able to take a look at me and see if he could help.

The neurosurgeon in Lafayette said that there was no way I would live through a trip from Lafayette to Shreveport, so Julian convinced him to drill a hole in my head to let out the pressure, which had been building since my arrival at the hospital. After completing this procedure, they got me on a plane to Shreveport, where my friend, Julian, met me.

One of the miracles in this story is the fact that there were only two neurosurgeons in the state of Louisiana capable of doing a surgery on a class five aneurysm, which is what I had. One was my good friend, Julian Bailes, and the other was Dr. Nanda from LSU medical school. Dr. Nanda was away at the time, which left my friend, Julian, as the only qualified neurosurgeon in the state at the time of this incident. Julian contacted Dr. Nanda by telephone and got temporary license to do the surgery with the assistance of another neurosurgeon.

After the surgery was completed and I was on life support in a drug-induced coma, the doctors were all having conversations about how I was not going to make it. It's been said that when someone is in a coma they can hear everything that's going on, and I'm here to tell you that's true. I heard every word they said. I heard one voice say, "You'd better go out there and prepare the family because this guy will never make it through this."

I then I heard my friend, Julian, respond by saying, "You don't know this guy. If anyone is going to make it through this, it's Edward Chauvin. And not only will he make it through, but he will make a one hundred percent recovery," and I was thinking: *That's my boy! Go Julian! That's my boy!*

(Let me go on record saying thank you to my good friend, Dr. Julian Bailes. I owe him so much.)

Shortly after that, I had a vision. In this vision, I was sitting in a chair and Jesus Christ was sitting in a chair across from me, just looking at me.

Now, Jesus does not look like any of the pictures that you have seen of Him in any traditional religion's books, magazines, or pictures. He's not this skinny-looking guy that has a feminine-looking face. He is a very masculine-looking man with a strong face, shoulder-length hair, and a full beard. But it's very well-manicured—very well kept.

It didn't feel like he was looking at me; it felt like he was looking inside of me. As Jesus looked at me, he said, "I have bigger and better things planned for you, Edward." And then I regained consciousness.

When I woke from the vision, it was actually the first time that I remember being awake, and when I came to, my good friend, Dr. George, was sitting on my bed.

"George, what are you doing here?" I asked.

"Ed, you ruptured a class five aneurysm in your head. Your family called me so I've come from California to see if I can help, but God's got bigger and better things planned for you."

I looked at him and I said, "Say that again, George. That's what Jesus just told me in my vision."

"What, that I came from California?" He didn't get what was happening at the time, or what I was referring to. He figured I was just rambling on, since I had just come out of a coma.

Dr. George Gonzalez is the founder of Quantum Neurology® and one of the top neurological specialists in the country. I was so blessed to have him right there for me, by my side. I don't remember much about when I first woke up, but I do know that he worked on me for several days. He told me later that when I regained consciousness, the left side of my body and the right side of my face were paralyzed and I couldn't move my arm or my body very well. There was a tube draining the fluid from my head, as well as an IV and other monitoring equipment hooked up to me. I was barely conscious, and fading in and out, as Dr. George and I tried desperately to connect with one another.

The first thing he established was that my vagal nerve stimulation—cranial nerves nine and ten, the nerves that control all the internal organs—was not working properly. These nerves are probably the most important ones to get rebooted and started up, because it promotes healing. He then did Quantum Neurology® with all of my myotomes, which are specific muscles coming off of the spine.

By next day, I was out of the ICU and in a new room. I was able to speak clearly and move both of my arms and legs. All the signs of paralysis in my face and body were gone. They had removed the drainage tube from my head, and—thank God and George—I was on the mend.

Dr. George continued to reintegrate my nervous system and just eleven days after my surgery, I walked out of the hospital on my own with no neurological deficits whatsoever. Finally, I was going home to be with my family.

The doctors had informed my family that I would need around-the-clock care for at least a year and it would be at least that long before I could even think about working, if I ever worked again. My family had called all of my office staff and told them that they'd better go find another job somewhere else because they didn't know when I would be coming back to work. My having this aneurysm had affected so many people's lives. It had affected the people working at my office, my family, and my children.

I feel so incredibly blessed, because what actually happened was this: twenty-nine days later, I went back to work full-time and have been practicing full-time ever since.

When you go through a traumatic event like that, people assume that you'll have long-term or short-term memory deficits. They feel sorry for you and worry about you. Even Sandra, one of my office staff who works with me on patients, said, "You know doc, I was really worried about your short-term and long-term memory loss, but when this one patient came in that you do a very specific procedure on—one that you don't do with anyone else—and you remembered to do it with her, I knew right then that you were back at a hundred percent."

After the patient left that day, I remember saying to Sandra, "You thought I had forgotten, didn't you?" She laughed and admitted that it was true. But she knew now that I was fully recovered with zero memory loss.

My Quantum Neurology® Experience

Nine years ago, I enrolled in a laser class and I was impressed by what a laser did as far as bringing back range of motion in a knee joint. I wanted to know everything about this laser and how to use it. Basically, all I knew about a laser was that if you put it on an arthritic knee, you got better range of motion to it. The guy who sold me the laser said, "I know a doctor that I highly recommend to teach you how to use your laser. His name is Dr. George Gonzalez and he teaches a course that I believe will answer all of your questions."

Soon after receiving the recommendation from the laser salesman, Dr. George was doing an event in Dallas, Texas. I went to that event and it changed the way I looked at the field of chiropractic by one hundred percent. When I returned to my office the next week, I put what he had taught us into practice right away. I was seeing one miracle after another. I was seeing people get full strength back to an arm or leg, full range of motion back to a shoulder or knee joint, back pain was going away instantly, and the list goes on and on. I thought to myself, *Wow, now this is the way to practice chiropractic!*

I continued to enroll myself in all of Dr. George's courses and when I finished his courses I believe I was the seventh Quantum Neurologist™ in the world. It's a high honor because we are seeing results that no other chiropractors are seeing. I thank God for Dr. George Gonzalez and what he has taught us in Quantum Neurology®.

I thank Dr. George for coming from California at my time of need and doing Quantum Neurology® on me. He got rid of the paralysis to the extent that I am now fully healed and neurologically sound. My body is fully functional and I am back to working out regularly. I don't lift four hundred pounds any more, but I do max out at three hundred, occasionally, to see if I can still do it. (I've been instructed by doctors not to lift extremely heavy weights any more, and I don't blame them for the recommendation.) I run about fourteen to sixteen miles per week on a treadmill. I can swim a mile without stopping. I can jump rope, lift things, and do whatever I want to do.

Since my recovery, and as a practicing Quantum Neurologist™, I see miracles of this magnitude on a regular basis. I feel fortunate to be alive and to be able to share with you not only my miracle, but the ones I've witnessed as well.

Chapter 2

From Above Down and From the Inside Out

Most people make their first visit to a chiropractor because they are in pain. Unfortunately, the pain alone doesn't usually get them to make the move to call a doctor; they usually wait until they get good and scared. The fear of their pain motivates them to do something about it. Using my thirty years of experience, I would venture to say that people usually wait somewhere between three to five weeks of trying home remedies, with no success, before they end up in my office.

It's really hard to treat people who have let themselves get to the point that they're in a wheelchair when they arrive at my office, but this happens over and over again. It's hard to get movement in the spine on someone who has waited this long to get treatment. If there is movement on the first visit, we can use Quantum Neurology® to take that movement and build a series of treatments to add further movement to other parts of the body.

I believe this works on both the physical and mental levels. The worry or fear a patient experiences are not the parts that I can heal. Worry, fear, and doubt actually detract from the treatment and can slow down the healing process considerably. People literally worry themselves sick. They become mentally paralyzed, doing nothing about their pain until they are afraid enough to do something about it. In the Bible, Jesus says, "Can any one of you by worrying add a single hour to your life?" (Matthew 6: 27 NIV) I think it's important to take this to heart because we all want quality of life, but we also want quantity of life. And that is what Quantum Neurology® and chiropractic delivers to people. We are not crisis care doctors, but rather, we are able to help people get healthy, and stay healthy, using natural methods.

Generally, people are only motivated by two things in life—one is fear and the other is desire, or love. If you took a plank, laid it down on the ground, and told someone that if they walked the plank to the end they'd find a twenty dollar bill there, most people would say, "I can do that easily," and they could because the desire to get the twenty dollar bill would be greater than the fear of walking the plank. However, if you took that same plank and laid it across two skyscrapers, the fear of heights in most people would be so great that they would say, "I'm not going to walk the plank for twenty dollars." In this case, their fear is actually greater than their desire and they would not walk the plank.

Now, let's take that situation where the plank was laid across two skyscrapers, and let's say that the person's child was on the other side of the plank and there was fire threatening to burn the child. Most people would fly across that plank, like it was nothing, and save their child. In this case, the love for the child is greater than the fear of heights. This scenario clearly shows that fear and desire are strong motivators to get people to respond and take action.

One simple truth about the human body is that it can heal itself, and it heals itself from above down and from the inside out. Let me explain what I mean by that. We have this innate ability to heal ourselves, and this is communicated through our nervous system from our brain, down the spinal cord, and out of the spine to the affected muscles, organs, and tissues, through the peripheral nervous system. This is an old chiropractic philosophy. We often say that interference of this communication, due to subluxations—or misalignments—of the spine, puts pressure on nerves, causing malfunction and pain in the body. Chiropractic has helped hundreds of thousands of cases like this by adjusting the spine to release these subluxations, thereby returning the patient to a normal state. This type of healing happens at such an amazing rate that it's unfathomable how many people we have affected.

Here's an example of how your ability to heal yourself happens from above down and from the inside out. If you cut your face and you cut your arm, your face will typically heal faster than your arm will. Or, if you cut your arm and your leg, your arm will heal quicker than your leg will. The reason this happens is because the life force that's generated by the brain and the spinal cord travels from above down and from the inside out.

Now this doesn't just pertain to physical healing, but it also pertains to mental and spiritual healing. People who are thinking the wrong way can actually have physical manifestations of pain that attack the body. It's all about resetting your thought process to affect the particular illness that is present.

Using spiritual principles, it can also be said that God affects us from above down and from the inside out. He doesn't work from the outside in and health doesn't come from the outside in. It comes from above down and from the inside out, through the nervous system. The communication in the body can be broken down into smaller transmissions, through the nervous system and the structure of the human body, in certain tissues of the body. Dr. George Gonzalez best demonstrates this in the science of Quantum Neurology®. We use red spectrum lasers and LEDs to turn on the signals of nerve transmission, which are not always caused by subluxations—or misalignments—of the spine causing nerve impingement.

This light energy is well communicated in the Bible in a few different ways. In Matthew 5:14, Jesus says, "You are the light of the world," and in Matthew 5:16, He says, "Let your light so shine before men that they may see your good works and glorify your Father in Heaven." You see, our bodies do communicate cellularly by light. It is the light energy that Jesus is speaking of that makes the communication and also allows healing to happen in the body. We don't think about our hearts beating and we don't think about breathing, but our bodies do those things automatically through the autonomic nervous systems. If you don't believe me, try holding your breath for about four minutes. If you hold your breath long enough, you're going to gasp for a breath of air. This reaction is innately present inside of your body; survival is ingrained in you.

In Ephesians 5:8, it says, "For you were once darkness, now you are light for the Lord. Live as children of light." This Scripture rings true for me because I have seen some amazing miracles happen in my office. I have seen people in wheelchairs who could move only one part of their bodies when they came into my office. They could move an arm or a leg and they had been that way for over twelve years. One had actually been that way for over twenty-two years. Using Quantum Neurology®, I was able to stimulate a nerve to get some movement into, first, a leg. Once the movement was established again, this allowed the nerves to regenerate themselves. Now these people are up and walking. I have one client, regularly walking two hundred fifty steps, who had been so paralyzed that she had to be strapped into her wheelchair. If she leaned to one side, she couldn't hold her body up; she would just fall off the chair. It was such an amazing process to see her core muscles start to work. Then we got her legs to start working and then her arms to start working better. Now she is walking and I thank God for it.

We are making progress in nerve rehabilitation through Quantum Neurology® with light therapy. There are so many new and exciting developments with this technology.

Many patients who come into my office are what I call, "mentally paralyzed." In other words, they will sit in their fear, doubt, and worry until they make themselves sick. They will go through all of this before they will make an appointment and come into my office to do something about it. This just blows my mind. It's a mental paralysis that causes them not to act. Their fear is greater than the motivation to come in. Their fear is greater than their desire to get well.

Our intention in Quantum Neurology® is to get people to understand that if you have a strong enough desire to get well, your body can—and will—heal itself. Given the right opportunities and the right communication between the brain and the cells and tissues of the body, your body tends to heal itself.

It's very important to bring awareness to the fuel that you put into your body. If you have an engine that isn't running well, you'll need to do repairs on the engine. If it is an engine that runs on gasoline and you mix in water with the gasoline, then the engine won't run very well at all. It may run a little bit but it will sputter and spark; it won't run like it's supposed to. The human body is just like the engine. If you put junk in, you'll get junky results. If you put good fuel in, you'll get great results. Your diet, and what you put in your body, is so important. In order for your body to heal itself, you'll need to put in the right fuel to aid the healing process and to encourage the right communication to your nervous system. This is done through chiropractic and Quantum Neurology®.

Growing up in a medically oriented family, I was programmed to believe that you didn't go to a medical doctor unless you were very sick. There is nothing wrong with seeing a medical physician, but we've been programmed into crisis care. I define crisis care as waiting until you have a crisis in your life to actually go to a doctor. Thank God for medical doctors. I would not be alive today to write this book if it had not been for my good friend, Dr. Julian Bailes, who did the surgery on my class five aneurysm.

After crisis care has been administered and the patient has made it through the crisis, there has to be a decision, on the patient's part, to take steps to keep the body healthy and to make decisions that move toward better health. I have created a list of five steps that will move you in the right direction toward a rich and healthy life. I will cover these five steps in the next chapter. I truly believe that no matter where you are, or how sick you are, if you follow these five steps instead of being paralyzed by fear, you will see and feel positive benefits and therefore live a more fruitful and abundant life.

Chapter 3

Genetics and Illness

Genetics play a part in every illness, but we cannot say that all sickness is caused by genetics. Otherwise, we would all be predestined, by our parents, as to how healthy or unhealthy we were going to be and what we were going to die of in this lifetime. Genetics, while important, are only responsible for twenty percent of our health; the other eighty percent is based on the daily choices we make. Therefore, choice becomes a huge factor in the equation. You can choose to do the right things or you can choose to do the wrong things.

In order to take a deeper look into how genetics work, we need to start from the beginning. In the beginning of life, a sperm and an egg unite to make a cell. That cell is called an undifferentiated cell, which means that it has no particular shape or characteristics to it. If you put that cell under a microscope, the only thing you can tell about it is that it's a human cell, unlike some of the differentiated cells that we're used to looking at in books and videos, such as blood cells, which are oval, red, and indented in the middle, or bone cells, which are kind of triangular. We've all seen pictures of nerve cells, which have a cell body with a long dendrite coming off of it. Most people know what those cells look like, but at the beginning of their development there is no universal shape or characteristic to cells.

Next, the cells divide into two, then four, then eight, sixteen, thirty-two, and sixty-four, and around the sixteenth day of life, a growth about as big as your thumbnail will form. This growth is called the morula, or blastula, which is not necessarily important for you to remember, but what is important is that at this point, the cells become differentiated cells; they start to take on shape or characteristics.

The first cells that differentiate in the body are the primitive brain and spinal cord. Why? The brain and the spinal cord coordinate all of the body's natural ability to exist. That is the first system to develop in the body, and the brain and nervous system is also the last system to die. For instance, when a person has a heart attack and their heart stops beating, they go to the hospital and the doctor resuscitates them to get their heart back to beating again. But when the brain is completely shut down, with no energy going through it, the person is declared dead. So the first system that is developed is the brain and spinal cord, and the last system to die is the brain and spinal cord. In other words, it is the key factor in development.

The next thing that happens in the embryological development of cells is that the cells begin to differentiate into bone tissue. These bone cells develop as a hard protective covering over the brain and spinal cord first. We call these the skull and the vertebra. And then arms form, and legs form, and ribs, and so forth, that start to protect other parts of the body.

Then, at the end of the nerve bundles, small buds begin to develop. The buds look just like the buds that you see on plants outside your home. But these buds don't turn into leaves or flowers or fruit; these buds turn into organs. And the first organs formed from these buds are the heart and circulatory system, which are equally as important as the nervous system.

Other buds turn into muscles and skin and other organs. The skin is actually the largest organ in the body. Most people don't think of the skin as a part of the body, or as an organ, but it is, just like the muscles of the neck and the back are organs.

The word of God says, "I will praise thee, for I am fearfully and wonderfully made. Marvelous are thy works, and that my soul knoweth right well." (Psalms 139:14) So where does all this life come from? In chiropractic and Quantum Neurology®, we call this life force "innate" which means "born within you." This innate life force is energy not similar to, but exactly like, electricity and light, and this electricity or light travels in the nervous system from above down and from the inside out by way of the nervous system. There are medical tests that prove the existence of this energy, and they are used every day in doctors' offices and hospitals all over the country. An EKG is a prime example. Looking at the graph of an EKG will show you the communication of the brain and the nervous system, and how it controls the heart and its contractions. From this information, a medical doctor can tell what is wrong with your heart and treat it appropriately. Another test that is done is an EMG, which stands for electromyography. This test shows how the transmission of a nerve impulse is communicating with the muscles supplied by that particular nerve. In other words, it shows how the nerve impulse transmission is sent to□ an arm, a leg, or some other part of the body.

Both EKG and EMG start with the letter "e," which stands for "electro." There is something not similar to, but exactly like, electricity, which travels to and from the nervous system from the brain, between every cell in your body. It travels from above down and from the inside out, and that is exactly how the body heals—from above down and from the inside out. Think about that one for a minute. If you get a cut on your face and your arm, your face will heal quicker than your arm will. If you get a cut on your arm and your leg, your arm will heal quicker than your leg will. The reason for this is that the electrical light transmission of the innate life force travels from above down and from the inside out, by way of the nervous system, and that's the way the body heals.

Think about it: a cut will heal from the inside before it heals on the outside. If it healed on the outside first, you'd call that an abscess, which is not a very good thing to have. That's why chiropractic Quantum Neurology® has become my chosen method of analysis and treatment of the human body. We're not taking away anything from the body or adding anything to the body, but allowing the body to recognize, and return to, normal function, using innate life force as the source of God-given ability. This is why chiropractic is so important in restoring normal function and communication to the entire body. If there is a subluxation (a misalignment of a vertebra, causing nerve pinching), then restoring vertebral alignment allows the body to return to homeostasis, or to normal function, by taking pressure off that nerve and therefore removing the deficit of that nerve.

In Quantum Neurology® chiropractic, Dr. George Gonzalez has made great breakthroughs in discovering the effects that light therapy has on the nervous system and the cells of the body to allow the body to heal itself. He has new concepts, which, when applied, can be one of the greatest ways of accessing this innate energy to work on a higher level of healing, using what God has already installed in each one of us. That's why chiropractic care has helped so many types of illnesses – not just sore backs and bones, lower back trouble, and neck problems. Chiropractic Quantum Neurology® is a system that communicates the brain's ability to the bodily functions and allows the body to function as it was designed to. While you have genetic tendencies toward certain factors in your life, you can function at the top, or the bottom, of your genetic potential.

I have a chart in my waiting room that shows how Chiropractic Quantum Neurology® can add years to life and life to years.

One of the things it says on the chart is, "died at forty—buried at sixty." I daresay no one wants that kind of life, but we can be fooled into just existing and not living.

In John 10:10, Jesus said, "The thief cometh not, but for to steal, and to kill, and to destroy: I am come that they might have life, and that they might have it more abundantly." These are choices we have to make for an abundant life. These choices are profound and simple. I would dare to say that no matter where you are as far as health or sickness, rather than being afraid and doing nothing it's better to take action steps to live at the top of your genetic potential, instead of the bottom of your genetic potential. You may ask yourself, *how can I do this?* I am happy to share with you what I believe is the answer to this question.

There are five things that influence your genetic potential:**Diet** – What you take into your body is so important.

Exercise – Without it you will lose your muscle mass and gain fat, and by age fifty or sixty, you may not be able to get out of your chair.

Proper Rest – We're supposed to get between six and eight hours of sleep a night but with our busy lifestyles, filled with information, sitting down all the time, analyzing everything, and not taking actions steps towards our health, we're losing the ability to rest, to have a deep REM sleep, and to wake up feeling energized again.

Freedom From Nerve Interference – Chiropractic and

Quantum Neurology® recognize this as the source for getting optimum nerve transmission for your body.

A Positive Mental Attitude – Thinking positive is very important to the body's function. If you are not thinking positively then you are thinking negatively. Negative thinking creates what we call psychosomatic disorders.

I've had a few cases where people's loved ones have died and they've been just devastated, and haven't been able to function in a normal capacity without those people in their lives. Sometimes this shows up as physical pain. In one of my patients, it showed up as right shoulder pain. We treated the patient and got the nerves of the spine functioning optimally, but the patient still had a tremendous amount of pain in his right shoulder.

After a series of inquiry questions, we discovered that his wife had passed away two years prior and he had loved his wife so much that he could not bear to live his life without her. He wouldn't go out of the house; he did nothing but sit around watching television and crying. We decided to show him a picture of his wife, and the minute we showed it to him he started to cry. Then we did a Quantum Neurology® technique in which we pulled the picture away from him to strengthen his response. This enabled his brain-body connection to allow for his wife leaving his life.

Immediately after doing this procedure, his shoulder pain level went from a grade of ten to a grade of zero within one visit. This man felt a freedom come over him that day and he started going out, engaging in activities, and enjoying his life again. His family came to me and asked, "What did you do to him? My God! He's a different person." I had to thank God because this powerful technique we had used made his nervous system strong enough that he could go out and function normally; he could live again.

In summation: Diet, exercise, proper rest, freedom from nerve interference and a positive mental attitude are the five key factors to living at the top of your genetic potential. Each of these will be covered in greater detail in the next chapter.

Chapter 4

Five Steps to Perfect Health

Why are you so worried about your health? Instead of worrying in fear, let's walk in faith. For the good book tells us that "without faith it is impossible to please God," (Hebrews 11:6) but it also says that "faith without works is dead," (James 2:26) meaning that it won't work for anyone. There are certain steps that you need to take to achieve good health. I have come up with what I believe to be the most important five.

Diet

Exercise

Proper Rest

Freedom From Nerve Interference

A Positive Mental Attitude

No matter what your health is like right now, you can take action to make it better…today. That's "now faith." The bible tells us that "now faith is the substance of things hoped for, the evidence of things not seen." (Hebrews 11:1) There are action steps that you have to take, with your faith in God, to get to where you want to go.

Diet

When we use the word "diet," that means *everything that you consume*. If you are a smoker, then you're consuming cigarette smoke into your body, and there's nothing that drains your body faster and more completely than smoking does, so I would strongly advise you to stop. It's one of the most positive things that you can do for yourself.

What other positive steps can you take?

There are hundreds, if not thousands, of diets out there. You can read about them on the internet until you're blue in the face. Some of them make a lot of sense, and they work for some people, but so many of them are focused on helping you lose weight, rather than getting you healthier than you are now and keeping you that way.

Much like everything else, my research of diets led me to the Bible. In the book of Leviticus, it tells you what to eat and what not to eat. I would think that the manufacturer of the human body—God Himself—would know exactly what you should put into your body and what you should take out of your body, so that's my reference.

God told the Jews not to eat leavened cakes, meaning, breads containing yeast. We're supposed to eat bread with no yeast in it, which would be unleavened bread. Yeast and funguses are causing most of the degenerative diseases that we see today, or are actually a part of those diseases. For example, diabetes, fungal infections, and a whole range of other problems are all caused by yeast and funguses in the diet. The more you leave those things out of your diet, the healthier it is for you to eat.

Sugar is also really bad for you. There should be no sugar in your diet whatsoever. It's poison. If you have to use a sweetener of some kind, I would highly recommend honey, preferably honey that is locally grown in the area where you live, as there are certain pollens in local nectar that actually bring health benefits to you.

If you're going to have grains in your diet and are going to make bread, use green-headed sprouted grains with no yeast. Ezekiel is a good brand of yeast-free, sprouted grain breads. In the book of Leviticus, it also tells us not to eat the fat or the blood of any animal. Now, in South Louisiana, where I'm from, they do double damage. They eat pieces of pork fat, called cracklings, which have the skin and the fat, and they taste delicious but they're actually terrible for you.

So, the Bible tells you not to eat fat and not to eat blood, but it doesn't tell you not to eat any animals. As a matter of fact, it's very specific; it says to eat animals that have split hooves and chew their cuds. Now, there are animals that have split hooves but don't chew their cuds, like pigs. We are not to be consuming pork at all. I know that in today's diet you'll probably eat some, but the less pork you can put into your body, the better.

Cattle (beef cows) have split hooves, they chew their cuds, and they are made to eat grass. Grass fed beef doesn't have the fat and marbling through the meat, like grain fed beef, and it is one of the healthiest meats that you can eat. So the Bible is true on that one. Lamb, goats, and deer also have split hooves and chew their cuds. All of these animals are Bible approved.

A horse does not have split hooves, so we shouldn't be eating horses. A camel has split hooves but doesn't chew its cud, so we shouldn't be eating camels either. Those animals that have split hooves and chew their cuds are good to eat and have health benefits to eating them. Stay away from pigs and animals with paws, like rabbits or squirrels.

When the Bible talks about eating animals and fish that come from the water, again, it's very specific; it says to eat fish that have fins and scales. So any fish that have fins and scales are okay for your body to consume. It's pretty simple.

Here in South Louisiana, they eat a lot of catfish. Catfish have fins but they have skin instead of scales. We should not be eating catfish because they are scavenger fish. They eat off the bottom and typically have a lot of pollution in them. Eating a lot of catfish has been known to cause health problems in the human body. So as much as you are able to, stay away from these foods and eat the ones that are healthy for you.

Certain birds are okay to eat but, again, the Bible is very specific as to which ones are to be eaten and which are not. I found it very interesting to read about this one in the good book. It says not to eat eagles. I personally don't know anyone who eats eagles but I'm sure there's somebody out there who does. It also says not to eat vultures. I wasn't surprised by that one; I wouldn't eat a vulture. And it also says not to eat hawks or ostriches. Not too many years ago, there was an emu population around South Louisiana and everyone was big into eating emus. Everyone was saying how great the meat was for you, but the Bible says not to eat ostriches and the emu is part of the ostrich family so I don't think we should be eating it.

The Bible also talks about insects. I personally don't eat any insects but there are insects listed in the Bible that you can eat. The insects that are Bible approved are ones with legs that have an actual hinge in the back legs. Those are okay to eat, so that means that grasshoppers are okay to eat. We don't eat too many grasshoppers here in Louisiana, but if you feel so inclined then go ahead and eat them.

The Bible talks about plants grown above the ground as being the best to eat. These include vegetables, tree bearing fruits, and tree bearing nuts. These are all good to eat. So let's get clear about some of these foods. According to what the Bible says, peanuts should not be eaten, as they are grown under the ground. Rice with bran on it can be consumed well by the human body, so we should be eating brown rice, not white rice. People in South Louisiana eat a lot of white rice.

Our bodies are made up of seventy-five percent water. This means that we should be consuming large quantities of water. Our bodies require us to drink eight to ten glasses of water a day for optimum health. Cola and other soft drinks do not count, and neither do any of those sports drinks for athletes. It's important to drink clean, pure water.

Exercise

Let's take a look at the health benefits of exercise. These benefits go beyond your genetic makeup because exercise is something you can do every day to improve your health. According to the Mayo Clinic, there are seven benefits to regular and consistent physical exercise. Exercise controls your weight; it can help prevent weight gain and help maintain weight loss, depending on what you consume in your diet. You don't need to set aside large chunks of time for exercise in order to reap the weight loss benefits, but it is very important for you to do some kind of exercise. The muscles of the body burn up more calories when you exercise, and when your body can't get the calories from your blood system, it goes to your fat and starts breaking your fat down into sugar that your body can use. So that's the way to get rid of fat and gain muscle, which is what you want. You want to have the strength without having the fat.

The second benefit to exercise is that it combats health conditions and diseases. No matter what your current weight is, being active boosts high-density lipoproteins (HDL's)—the good cholesterol—and decreases the unhealthy triglycerides. This is a one-two punch that keeps your blood flowing smoothly and decreases the risk of cardiovascular disease. In fact, regular physical activity can help you prevent or manage a wide range of health issues and concerns, including strokes, type 2 diabetes, depression and certain types of cancer and arthritis. It's also harder for you to fall if you're physically active and in good shape, so I recommend that you exercise on a daily basis. Exercise also improves your mood. Physical activity stimulates various brain chemicals that may leave you feeling happier and more relaxed. You may also feel better about your appearance and yourself when regular exercise is obtained, which can boost your confidence and improve your self-esteem.

Regular physical activity can improve your muscle strength and boost your endurance. Exercise and physical activity deliver oxygen and nutrients to your tissues to help your cardiovascular system work more efficiently. When your heart and lungs are more efficient, you have more energy to go about your everyday chores, so you enjoy your life even more.

Exercise also helps you to sleep better. Regular physical activity can help you fall asleep faster and sleep deeper. Just don't exercise too close to your bedtime because the exercise boosts your metabolism, which doesn't allow you to go to sleep right away. We recommend that you exercise either in the morning or in the afternoon.

Exercise can also put the spark back into your sex life. Regular physical activity can leave you feeling energized and looking better, which may have a positive effect on your sex life. It can also lead to enhanced arousal for women, and men who exercise regularly are less likely to develop erectile dysfunction than men who don't exercise.

Exercise can be fun. It gives you a chance to unwind and enjoy the outdoors, or simply engage in activities that make you happy. There's nothing like a good game of volleyball, softball, tennis, or any activity you enjoy doing that keeps you physically fit.

Proper Rest

According to recent studies, human beings need six to eight hours of sleep per night. Some people get this much sleep each night and some people don't. Perhaps the people who don't get enough sleep could use some tools or ideas to help them make a better choice. I'd like to share nine tips on how to get six to eight hours of sleep per night, without taking medication or drugs, and it won't cost you a dime to implement these things. What they will do is help to keep you in the right perspective to get the amount of sleep you need.

Tip #1 – Stick to a Schedule

It's funny that we train our kids to get the proper amount of rest and yet we don't follow what we teach them ourselves. We say things like, "its nine o'clock, time for bed. We have to make sure that you are rested so you can have a good day at school tomorrow." Then we stay up until midnight watching television and wonder why we can't sleep when we turn off the TV. You see, what we are teaching the children is a really great habit to form. If we went to bed when we put them to bed, we would also get enough sleep to have a great day the next day. It's the habit of going to bed at a regular time every night that gets your brain chemistry ready to sleep at that time. Neurologically, you can train yourself to become sleepy at a certain time and by doing so you'll have a deep and restorative sleep.

Tip #2 – Sleep Only at Night

You may say, "I like to sleep in the daytime," but sleeping during the daytime actually messes up the rhythm of sleep at night. It doesn't allow you to get a full night of sleep because you've had rest in between. Your mind and your body will believe that you've already had the sleep you needed, and will make it harder for you to get the deep REM sleep needed to wake up feeling rested and restored.

Tip #3 – Exercise Regularly

Not only does exercise have health benefits but it can also help you get that all-important deep night of sleep. Your body uses the time you sleep to recover its muscles and joints that have been exercised. Twenty to thirty minutes of exercise daily can help you sleep better. Just be sure not to exercise right before you go to bed. It's important to exercise early in the morning or in the afternoon because exercise stimulates the body. Aerobic activity right before you go to bed will keep you from being able to go to sleep. It will actually wind you up instead of winding you down for a good night's sleep.

Tip #4 – Take a Hot Bath or Shower Before Going to Bed

Another valuable tip for creating a restful sleep is to take a hot bath or shower right before you go to bed. This will allow all of your tense muscles to relax, which then allows your mind to relax into a deep and restful night's sleep.

Tip #5 – Avoid Eating Food Right Before Going to Bed

It's so important not to eat food right before you go to bed. I would highly recommend that you allow two-and-a-half hours from the time you eat until the time you lay down to go to sleep. It takes that long for your stomach to digest the food that you've eaten. The digestion process activates and stimulates other parts of your body, so eating right before you lay down to go to sleep is a set up for a less-than-fantastic night of sleep. Your stomach will be gurgling and moaning, and that alone might keep you up. Allowing two-and-a-half hours for your food to digest gives those parts of your body a chance to rest while you sleep.

Tip #6 – Avoid Caffeine

Drinking coffee, soda, tea, or anything with caffeine at night will surely interrupt your sleep pattern. If the coffee is strong, you may feel more like going for a jog, cleaning the house, or watching a movie than lying down and going to sleep.

Tip #7 – Read a Book

There's something really powerful about reading a good book right before you go to bed. It's nighttime and because you have set up a regular time for sleep every night, your body knows that sleep is coming very soon. You start reading your book, your eyes start to droop, and you feel like you can drift off any time into sleep. Once you close the book and lay down, your mind will continue to think about what you were reading and you'll fade off into a nice, deep sleep. You may even dream about what you were reading, so make sure the book isn't something really intense, violent, or upsetting to your mind.

Tip #8 – Keep Your Bedroom Slightly Cooler Than the Rest of Your Home

Keeping your bedroom slightly cooler than the rest of your home is a powerful tip for you. This wouldn't even occur to most people but think about it: if you wear pajamas when you sleep, you've climbed into a warm set of clothing and then into a nice, warm bed. If your room is also warm, you may find yourself waking up hot, or in a sweat, in the middle of the night. Keeping the room a little cooler balances this and increases your chances of a restful night of sleep.

Tip #9 – Sleep in Silence

As much as you are able to, sleep in silence. Many people like to sleep with the television on or with music blasting, but this is not supportive of a good night's sleep in any way. The most important part of sleeping is allowing your body and mind to rest. Your mind gets wound up by television and music, and will continue to stay active if you have those on while you're attempting to sleep. It is in your best interest to turn off all the noises of the outside world and tune in to the inside world before you go to sleep. Lay down in silence, take some nice, deep, relaxing breaths, and ease yourself into a restful sleep.

And there you have it. Those are my nine tips to getting proper rest without taking any medications or drugs.

Freedom From Nerve Interference

Using chiropractic and Quantum Neurology® techniques has brought me much success in relieving unwanted nerve interferences that people have had. I believe that a hundred percent of the population need chiropractic Quantum Neurology® treatments. Not just the people who have aches and pains, and the people who are not feeling quite right, but a hundred percent of the people. Why? Because there are subluxations of the spine that cause nerve interference, as we discussed in an earlier chapter, and because the nervous system is the most important system of the body. It's the first developed, and the last to die, so it therefore stands to reason that taking care of that system by making regular maintenance visits to your chiropractic Quantum Neurologist™ is very important.

There are things that you can do to help. For instance, having good posture gives you some degree of neurological control over your life. When people are bent over, they start to pinch off the neurological system to the rest of the body and have health problems because of it, or aches and pains related to it.

But there's more to it than just pinched nerves caused by misalignments—or subluxationsof the spine. There is also interference of the mind, the cranial nerves, and the organs, which can be helped through chiropractic Quantum Neurology®. There are nerve-muscle connections, called myotomes, and nerve-skin connections, called dermatomes, all of which originate from the spine. Every organ in the body is connected to the spine in this way. Chiropractic is the study of how these particular nerves exit the spine and connect to these particular tissues to give you life, health, and function. If a vertebra is misaligned and is squeezing, or putting pressure on, a nerve, it can alter the transmission of that nerve to the muscle, to the organ, and to the skin or the tissues that it supplies in the body. That's why some people say, "I didn't go to the chiropractor because I didn't have any pain." The truth is that nerve interference goes way beyond pain levels. Pain is primarily what brings people into our office and, of course, we do recommend that people come in when they are in pain. But there are also nerve interferences caused by the mind and Dr. George Gonzalez addresses these in Quantum Neurology®.

I remember in chiropractic college we studied the cranial nerves in the head to make sure that people didn't have a concussion, a brain tumor, or something that would lead to a referral out of our office. At that time, I had no idea we'd be helping so many people with nerve interferences to these cranial nerves. For example, if your eyes are not functioning in all four quadrants, we look to the specific cranial nerves that control those movements.

Quite often in sports injuries or in falls or random accidents, not only do people break arms and legs and maim themselves, but these cranial nerves get distorted. Why is that so important? Well, you can fix the breaks in the arms and the legs through crisis care and traditional medical treatments, but after that these cranial nerves have never been fixed. Quantum Neurology® addresses that and by using light therapy, we are able to get the nerves functioning optimally again. This restores better eyesight control to the patient who was in the accident.

Cranial nerves are said to be responsible for ADHD and ADD, which we see often in children. Usually the signs of cranial nerve damage in children are evident because they were doing well in school and then had some type of accident or severe illness. Since their cranial nerves weren't functioning well, their grades plummeted. Perhaps they were getting A's and B's and now are down to making D's and F's. We have helped quite a few patients like these in my office and brought these children back to getting straight A's and B's again. It's so freeing to see this type of recovery happen right before your eyes, and thanks to Quantum Neurology® it's not only possible, but is happening every day, all over the country.

A Positive Mental Attitude

The Bible says, "As a man thinketh in his heart, so is he." (Or as a woman thinketh in her heart, so is she.) (Proverbs 23:7) What this means is that the power of positive thinking is directly connected to our ability to remove, control, and eliminate negative thoughts. This is so important because if you are thinking the wrong way, you will speak the wrong way. The Bible says that if you speak the wrong way, that's where your ship will head. It says your ship will head in the direction that your tongue tells it to go. (James 3:4-5) This means that what we speak is what happens in our lives. Notice how much this is true. Those who speak of being sick continue to be sick. Those who speak of poverty, on a regular basis, continue to be money poor. Those who go around saying, "life is good" all the time usually have a good life. So where it's important to think positive thoughts, it's equally important to *say* positive thoughts. Doing this will directly affect the outcome of your life.

What, exactly, are negative thoughts? We will define negative thoughts as doubt, fear, worry, doom and gloom, and the constant focus on what could go wrong in your life. These are clear signs of negative thinking.

When I was being raised, our parents taught us that God is a good God and that God wants to give good things to you. But it's important to take action with your faith to get to where God wants you to be. In other words, pleasing God by your faith is great but pleasing God by your actions is better. People hear what you say but they notice what you do even more than what you say. I truly believe that thinking positively is one of the most powerful things you can do to have a good life.

I heard a story about this that really affected me and the way I think, and I'd like to share it with you.

Imagine you have two glasses filled with mud and this mud represents all the negative thoughts that have been playing out in your life ever since you were a child. You really want to get those thoughts out of your mind and start having more positive experiences, but the mud has been in those glasses for such a long time that it has dried up and turned to a solid form and it's really stuck in there.

You take the first glass of mud and bring it to a psychotherapist. The doctor says, "I want to take you back to your childhood and we'll discuss all the negative things that happened to you in your life." As you do this, you start chipping away at the mud with a metal spoon and scooping it out of the glass. When all the mud is out of the glass, you thank the doctor and go back to your life. But you notice that the glass is still dirty and now it's empty as well, and you wonder how you'll keep the glass from getting filled up with mud all over again.

With the second glass of mud, you decide to try something different. You begin replacing all those negative thoughts from your childhood with positive thoughts, and as you do this you hold the glass under a faucet and turn the faucet on. You watch as the water turns the hard, dried up mud into wet, liquid mud. As the water continues to flow into the glass, the liquid mud begins to overflow out of the glass and soon the dirty water is completely replaced, leaving you with a clean glass filled with clear water. There is no longer any sign of mud having been in the glass.

I believe this is a metaphor for our lives. The more we fill our glass with water (positive thoughts), the more mud (negative thoughts) will be replaced until we end up with a glass full of clear liquid (a healthy, happy life). For this purpose, I highly recommend that you read positive articles and books. I believe the word of God is the place to start. When you read the Bible, you'll find that it is full of positive stories and thoughts that will impact your life forever.

You may also want to watch positive programs. This can be tough to do with all of the news and negative shows on the air these days. If you do watch the news, make sure that you watch something positive immediately after watching the news. Watch positive television shows, think positive thoughts, and speak positive words and soon you will have the life that you are looking for.

I have shared in this chapter what I believe are the five most powerful steps you can take to achieve good health. No matter how healthy or unhealthy you are at this point in your life, if you learn these five steps and you do them your life and health will improve dramatically.

Chapter 5

Living Healthy Without Spending a Fortune

One of the most important keys to obtaining good health is a positive mental attitude. We are not sick people trying to get well; we are well people fighting off sickness. I think this is something very important to remember.

In the Bible, after God had told His people all about His blessings and the curses that would fall upon them if they didn't do what He told them to do, He said this, "I call heaven and earth to record this day against you, that I have set before you life and death, blessing and cursing: therefore choose life, that both you and your children may live." (Deuteronomy 30:19) So, choosing good health is an obtainable goal with God and women and men. You can choose to think positively and make a plan. Creating this plan is free, but will cost you some time to prepare.

Take an Inventory

A great exercise you can do is to take an inventory of your life and health, and keep it positive. When you look at where you are currently compared to what you'd like your health to be like, it can sometimes seem impossible. "With God all things are possible." (Matthew 19:26) Whether you currently have health problems or just a desire to have better health, focusing on your problems will make better health seem to be miles away. But remember this: a mile is a trial, a yard is still hard, but an inch is a cinch.

Now go and get a blank piece of paper and come back to do this powerful process. (A piece of paper doesn't cost much but when you complete this process you will find much value on that page.)

Draw a line down the middle of the page, from top to bottom. In the top left corner of the page, I want you to write a zero. In the top right corner, I want you to write a ten. Over the middle line at the top of the page, write the number five. I've promised to share with you ways to achieve better health without spending a lot of money, and in order to do this I'd like you to answer the following questions for me.

When it comes to your health…

Do you want to be a ten or do you want to be a five?

Would you rather be a five or a three?

Or do you want to be a zero?

Most people, if they have any sense at all, will choose to be a ten (the best that they can be).

Let's start by taking inventory and creating your plan. Take an inventory of all the things you do and rate them using the following examples as your guide.

In my opinion, reading the Bible is a very positive thing to do. If you do read the good book, you can put "read the bible" on the right side of the page in the five through ten category because it's something that moves you toward the positive. You can read God's word concerning health, love, forgiveness, or strength to give you creative ideas and then start acting upon them. Doing this will bring you closer to your ten and closer to better health.

Here's another example. If you are a cigarette smoker, write that down on the left side of the page, since that is an unhealthy choice. It would qualify in the category of five to zero.

If you eat a lot of salads, put that on the right side of page. If you eat a lot of fatty foods, like French fries or potato chips, put that on the left side of the page.

If you eat a lot of sugar, carbohydrates, and junk food, put those down on the left side of the page. They are clearly unhealthy choices.

Some choices may not be as obvious as others. For instance, your posture is very important to your neurological function. Having good posture costs you nothing. It's as easy as sitting up straight, standing up straight, and, more importantly, making a clear decision to bring awareness to using your postural muscles. So if you're sitting properly, that would be something you'd put on the right side of the paper because it's about bettering your health and bringing better neurological function.

On the flip side, if you're sitting in a recliner with your feet up and your head pushed forward, that would be something you would write on the left side of the page. I know people who sleep in a recliner, and that would be considered a very unhealthy choice because it takes your spine and puts it in an abnormal posture, which molds your spine in an undesirable way. It also diminishes the neurological flow from your neck, down your back, to your hips, joints, legs, arms, and elbows, right down to your fingertips. This qualifies as a negative choice, in my opinion.

If you exercise, put that on the left side. I highly recommend that you exercise at least four times a week for at least thirty to forty minutes. This will get your blood going and your circulatory system flowing. It will work out your heart and other muscles. There are many ways to work out for free with no gym membership needed. You can walk, bicycle, and swim. When it comes to moving your body, just do the things that feel easy and natural to you.

Another thing that you can do to stay healthy is to laugh. Laugh out loud as much as possible, as laughter increases the activity of the brain in a way that brings healing. As a matter fact, the Bible says, "A merry heart doeth good like a medicine." (Proverbs 17:22) Laughing regularly helps your attitude, your psychic makeup, and it helps the organs inside your body to function better.

The Mirror Technique

Another thing you can do that would end up on the right side of your paper is an exercise I like to call, "the mirror technique." This exercise is great because it doesn't cost one penny to do. Everyone has at least one mirror in their house and most people have the ability to talk to themselves. Coupling these two things together is all you need to do the mirror technique. It's quite simple: just look into the mirror and tell yourself positive things about yourself. For example, "I am capable of anything that comes my way today. I am well able to do this task that I am setting out to do. I am getting better looking every day. In every way I'm getting better and better. I am strong, powerful, and capable. I am worthy of everything good. I choose to live a healthy lifestyle."

Over time, these affirmative thoughts, spoken out loud to yourself in the mirror, will not only help you to create a better self-image but will teach your subconscious mind to think that way, without effort. This technique brings focus to the good in us, instead of always focusing on negative thoughts. Let's face it, we all have negative thoughts and they don't do us any good at all. They certainly don't support a healthy way of living or being. In the Bible, it tells us that Satan comes to steal, kill, and destroy. But Jesus came to give us life and to give it to us more abundantly. (John 10:10) Jesus wants us to feel good about ourselves and so we honor Him when we do the mirror technique and think positively. Prayer is also a good choice, and one that I would put on the right side of the page as well.

Drinking soft drinks, instead of water, would be a left side choice.

Eating candy, instead of a meal, also goes on the left of the page.

Procrastination is a left side choice. Why put off until tomorrow what you can do today?

As soon as you finish this chapter, set this book down and start the process. Take your inventory. Get your piece of paper and go through all the areas discussed in the previous chapter. List your positive and negative habits on the page.

Look at your diet and list diet choices you make (as many as you can think of)

Look at your exercise choices and write those down

Your freedom from nerve interference (remember, this includes your posture)

Proper rest (think about all the tips I have given you)

Positive mental attitude (consider building this using this inventory exercise, the word of God, and the mirror technique)

The Healing Power of Forgiveness

Another tip I'd like to share with you, in regard to building a healthy mental way of being, is the power of forgiveness. For optimum health, I think it's important for you to forgive everyone who has ever hurt you. I know that may not be an easy one for you. I understand you may have had a lot of hurtful things happen in your life…I sure have. But God wants you to forgive these people, not just for them, but to set yourself free.

I laughed out loud when a counselor shared this with me some years back. Something had happened to me that felt really bad and I was extremely angry at the person who did it. I was so angry with them that I just wanted them out of this world. I shared this with the counselor, Dr. Jeff Sandoz, and he told me that he'd like me do something for him as an exercise. He challenged me to get on my knees every morning and pray for that person I had wished ill upon. He told me to pray that this person would have all the health, happiness, and prosperity that I prayed and wished for myself.

As I laughed out loud at him, I said, "Jeff, you don't understand…I want these people dead!" Again, he challenged me to do the process for two weeks. "God's going to know that I'm lying," I told him.

"Just do it anyway," was his response. I promised him I would.

The next morning, even though I felt pretty stupid, I got on my knees and started to say the prayer that Dr. Jeff had told me to say. I prayed for that person to have all the health, happiness, and prosperity that I wanted for myself. A strange thing happened and it didn't even take two weeks of me doing it every day.

The first time I did it, I almost laughed my way all the way through it. That's how insincere I was about it and how much I thought it wouldn't work. I figured that God knew I was lying so He wouldn't even listen to the prayer. But God listens to all prayers and through my obedience to the word of God, He started to change my heart from the inside out. Before the two weeks were over, I started to feel so sorry for those people that I knelt down and cried for them. Of course, my praying didn't take away what they had done to me, but it did take away the anger that I had for them in my heart. It helped to set me free from the upset and anger. My wishing harm on them only hurt me; it didn't hurt them in any way. I was the only one who was feeling the ill effects of my disdain for them and what they had done.

Forgiveness is very important to a healthy mind and body. Choose to love. Choose to love as much as possible. Love others and love yourself. You may feel like saying, "Dr. Chauvin, you don't understand. I can't love these people. They did me wrong. I can't do it." If this describes what you're feeling right now, I'd like to share something with you. I heard it some time ago and it really helps me.

Just to be able to stand in the same room as someone who has hurt you, and not try to hurt them back, is a form of love.

When I heard this, I thought to myself, *I can do that.*

Take it one step at a time. Inch by inch, step by step, forgive yourself for judging others and forgive yourself for judging yourself. It's all a process. Start where you're at because without forgiveness it's impossible to love yourself, and you must love yourself before you can love others.

Forgiveness is a right side activity. For each person you forgive, add that to the right side of your inventory list. God says that "obedience is better than sacrifice." (1 Samuel 15:22) Being obedient to God, and doing what He said to do in the good book, changed me in less than two weeks. This will work for anyone because "God is no respecter of persons." (Acts 10:34) If He did it for me, He'll do it for you.

Doing the techniques I have shared with you in this chapter will help your body's and mind's way of being. Making right sided choices toward the good, and toward God, will increase the betterment of your health. This is far more powerful than making left sided choices, such as hate, anger, or getting even with someone who you think has done you wrong. Those choices are never good for anyone.

Can Do

You are a "can do" person, not a "can't do" person. A can't do person goes around saying, "I can't do this." This is what I'd call a left sided choice. It falls on the left side of your inventory chart for sure. I live in America and I am an American. If you look at the word American, you'll see that it ends with the letters I-C-A-N. It doesn't say, "I can't," it says, "I can." The Bible says, "I can do all things through Christ who strengthens me." (Philippians 4:13) But how can He strengthen you if you don't follow his ways?

Making these choices is very important:

Forgive
Think positive thoughts

I understand that sometimes when you look at where you are and where the current state of your health is, it can seem impossible to imagine it being any other way. I get that. I would encourage you to remember that "with God all things are possible." (Matthew 19:26) I've seen it time and time again. You can call it "God" or you can call it whatever you like to call it. I just know it works. I've seen so many miracles in my time that, at this point, it is impossible for me *not* to believe in miracles.

Sing, Sing, Sing

Here's another thing you can do to better your health without spending a fortune: sing. Sing to yourself, to God, or to someone you love, but sing! It doesn't cost you anything and it creates positive results in your state of good health. It's impossible to sing and be angry at the same time. Isn't that great? You can sing, be happy, give praises to God, and improve your health, all at the same time.

Stretch Your Body

Stretching is another key to good health. It takes about a minute per muscle, it's free, and the health benefits are incredible. If we all stretched our muscles every day, we'd have a lot fewer physical problems. In order to stretch a muscle properly, you have to stretch that muscle for a full minute.

When I was growing up, I remember doing warm-up exercises in school. They would have us reach over for ten seconds, switch legs, and repeat. Sometimes they would have us bouncing up and down on a muscle and they had the nerve to call that "stretching." That's really not a stretch at all.

To do a proper stretch is to cause elongation of that muscle into the fullest range of motion that you can put that joint and muscle through. The best way to get the benefits of stretching your muscles is to put a clock in front of you so you can see exactly how long you have stretched for. Stretching for fifteen seconds is really not a stretch at all. A fifteen second stretch will actually cause the muscle to tighten. It preloads the muscle so there is a bit of a benefit, but if you want the full benefit then stretch for a minute per muscle.

So, what are the benefits of a good stretch?

Stretching increases the range and motion of your joints.

Stretching reduces muscle tension. If you're experiencing stress in your life, try stretching, as it reduces tension. As you stretch, you will feel the stress lighten up.

Stretching enhances muscular coordination. We all need coordination. The older you get, the more coordination you need to keep you from falling and getting injured.

Stretching increases the circulation of blood to various parts of your body. Stretching is so good for your body! In Quantum Neurology®, we know that each muscle, or myotome, is supplied by a coordinated nerve and each myotome has an associated organ. So by stretching a muscle, you're not only causing the blood supply to that muscle to be better but you're bringing better energy to the organ that the muscle supplies. This allows the organ to become stronger as well.

Stretching increases energy levels. We all need more energy to get through the day and to thoroughly enjoy our lives.

Stretching is good for people of all ages and should be done every day. Everyone can learn to stretch, regardless of age or flexibility. There are guidelines for stretching safely. If you've never stretched before, make sure you get instructions on how to do it safely and carefully. You can type "how to stretch my muscles" into an online search engine and I'm sure you'll find thousands of results. If you belong to a gym, the instructors will be glad to teach you. There may even be a specific course on stretching, so check your course schedule at the gym.

Drink Water

Another cost-effective way to improve your health is to drink water. I keep mentioning that, don't I? I keep saying it because it's that important. So many people are walking around dehydrated, feeling sick, and they don't know why. Most headaches are caused by dehydration.

The human body is made up of about seventy-five percent water. The daily recommendation for water consumption is eight eight-ounce glasses of water per day (depending on age, gender, and amount of body fat). Most people don't drink enough water and they wonder why they feel off. Some may think that they are drinking enough liquid because they drink soda-pop, coffee, power drinks, sports drinks, or fruit juices all day long. None of those are water. I'm here to tell you that these don't count and many of them actually dehydrate you more. Sports drinks are high in sugar and minerals, which can be good for some athletes during the course of a heavy, sweat-breaking workout, but sitting around drinking them is not good for the body. It's very important for your body to get good, clean, pure water.

In the course of a typical day, you will breathe, sweat, and urinate. You'll need to drink a substantial amount of water just to replace what leaves your body during these routine processes. If you're not drinking enough water, you'll feel thirsty all day long and your urine will be brownish or even bright yellow. If you are drinking enough water, you'll rarely feel thirsty and you'll produce a lot of very clear or very light yellow urine. These are clues that you are drinking the right amount of water.

What type of water should you drink?

Regular tap water can be full of chlorine and fluoride. These types of minerals are added to water, typically in big cities, and can be toxic and harmful to your body. I highly recommend drinking filtered water or bottled water. My personal favorite is Aquafina®. I love the taste of it. We tested it and I think it's one of the cleanest waters you can drink. So if you can find Aquafina®, do so. This isn't a commercial for Aquafina®. I get no kickbacks or compensation from them, I just like their water. There are other good waters out there too.

Eat a Healthy Breakfast

Another tip for good health that won't cost you a fortune is eating a good breakfast. For years, I've been questioning patients who come in my office and it's amazing how few people actually eat breakfast. A healthy breakfast is the cornerstone of a good diet. The energy from a healthy breakfast can carry you through your morning and aid you in making healthier choices throughout the day, such as choosing not to drink coffee or eat sweets. Studies have shown that eating a healthy breakfast lowers cholesterol. I know that probably doesn't seem possible but most of the breakfast foods eaten, like oatmeal or whole grain breads and cereals, are high in fiber. Fruit is also good.

Think, for just a moment, about not eating breakfast. Your body has been asleep for seven or eight hours, then you wake up and go about your day. By the time you eat your lunch, around noon, it's been ten to sixteen hours since you put any food into it. Your body doesn't have the fuel it needs, so it goes into starvation mode. Next, your metabolism starts to shut down. It takes the calories that you have as sugars in your body and turns them to fat.

What we want is less fat and more muscle. If you are not going to eat a full breakfast, at least eat some protein at breakfast time to give your body some fuel.

Multi-Vitamin/Multi-Mineral Supplements

I take a multi-vitamin/multi-mineral supplement every morning. Some people believe that if they take a vitamin or mineral supplement, they can eat anything else they want throughout the day. This type of thinking is counter-productive. If you are not eating whole, healthy foods and you're taking a vitamin, thinking that you're doing something healthy, you're really fooling yourself. In this situation, the supplements are just counteracting the carcinogens that you're putting into your body. This is like fighting a losing battle. I highly recommend that you eat a good breakfast, take your multi-vitamin/multi-mineral supplement, and eat healthy, whole foods the rest of the day. This will set you up for optimum health.

Physical Touch

Physical touch is important to good health. Studies done in the 1930s in orphanages showed that infants who were touched, picked up, or nuzzled thrived and grew faster than those who were left alone in their cribs. Human touch is healing to the soul. This is another reason why people should go see chiropractors. Even if you are not in a relationship or in a touchy-feely family, at least you'll be touched by your doctor, which can bring healing to your body.

Eat Fruits and Vegetables

I'm sure it will not surprise anyone when I say that eating fruits and vegetables is a very important part of a healthy diet. If you're able to eat organic fruits and vegetables, it's even better. Eating fruits and vegetables actually fights cancers and carcinogens in the body. The phytonutrients that you receive from eating fruits and vegetables are an important part of creating a healthy lifestyle. Eating healthy, organic fruits and vegetables has been shown to improve the health of people with heart conditions, cancer, type 2 diabetes, and the list goes on and on.

A Small Amount of Sunlight Each Day

Another thing you can do to improve your health is to get a small amount of sunlight, each and every day. If you get about ten minutes of sunlight each day at noon, your body will produce somewhere between ten thousand and twenty-five thousand international units of vitamin D. If you tried to get that much vitamin D from drinking milk, you'd have to drink twenty-five to sixty quarts a day. Why not stand out in the sun for ten minutes at noon time?

Vitamin D is vital to creating and maintaining strong and healthy bones. Vitamin D deficiency can cause muscle weaknesses, as well as dozens of internal types of cancers, multiple sclerosis, and type 1 and type 2 diabetes. We highly recommend ten minutes of sun each day. There is no reason to use sunscreen, as long as you're only doing the ten minutes recommended.

On the flip side, it's important not to get too much sun or get sunburned. We all know that long periods of sun exposure will cause skin problems. So stick to the ten minutes to produce the vitamin D that you need for strong bones and joints.

Daily Physical Activities

Daily physical activity is an important part of a healthy lifestyle. Walking for fifteen minutes a day won't cost you a dime. You don't have to join a health club to take a hike or a nice walk down the road. Doing sit-ups and push-ups doesn't require any special equipment either. You can stay strong and healthy by doing these particular physical activities daily.

Stay the Course

I can't tell you how many people sit down, make a list of better healthy choices, stick to the plan for a while, and then quit right before getting the result they were working so hard to create. It's important to finish what you start and more important, to your overall health, to continue what you started for the rest of your life.

I want to end this chapter by sharing a poem that is very important to me. It is right in alignment with the way I think and how I suggest others think as well.

The Race

"Quit! Give up, you're beaten!"
They did shout and plead,
"There's just too much against you now
this time, you can't succeed."
And as I start to hang my head
in front of failure's face.
My downward fall is broken
by the memory of a race.

And hope refills my weakened will
as I recall that scene.
For just the thought of that short race
rejuvenates my being.
A children's race, young boys, young men,
now I remember well.
Excitement, sure, but also fear;
it wasn't hard to tell.

They all lined up so full of hope,
each thought to win that race.
Or tie for first, or if not that,
at least take second place.
And fathers watched from off the side,
each cheering for his son.
And each boy hoped to show his dad
that he would be the one.

The whistle blew and off they went,
young hearts and hopes of fire.
To win, to be the hero,
that was each young boy's desire.
And one boy in particular,
his dad was in the crowd.
Was running near the head and thought,
"My dad will be so proud."

But as he speeded down the field
across a shallow dip,
The little boy who thought to win,
lost his step and slipped.
Trying hard to catch himself,
his hands flew out to brace,
And mid the laughter of the crowd,
he fell flat on his face.

So down he fell and with him hope.
He couldn't win it now.
Embarrassed, sad, he only wished
to disappear somehow.
But as he fell his dad stood up
and showed his anxious face,
Which to the boy so clearly said,
"Get up and win the race!"

He quickly rose, no damage done,
behind a bit, that's all,

And ran with all his mind and might
to make up for his fall.
So anxious to restore himself,
to catch up and to win,
His mind went faster than his legs,
he slipped and fell again.

He wished that he had quit before
with only one disgrace.
"I'm hopeless as a runner now,
I shouldn't try to race."
But in the laughing crowd he searched
and found his father's face,
That steady look that said again,
"Get up and win the race".

So he jumped up to try again
ten yards behind the last.
"If I'm to gain those yards," he thought,
"I've got to run real fast."
Exceeding everything he had,
he regained eight or ten.
But trying so hard to catch the lead,
he slipped and fell again.

Defeat! He lay there silently,
a tear dropped from his eye.
"There's no sense running anymore.

Three strikes I'm out, why try?"
The will to rise had disappeared,
all hope had fled away.
So far behind, so error prone, a
loser all the way.

"I've lost, so what's the use?" he thought,
"I'll live with my disgrace."
But then he thought about his dad,
who soon he'd have to face.
"Get up!" an echo sounded low,
"Get up and take your place!"
"You were not meant for failure here,
get up and win the race!"

So far behind the others now,
the most he'd ever been.
Still he gave it all he had
and ran as though to win.
Three times he'd fallen stumbling,
three times he'd rose again.
Too far behind to hope to win,
he still ran to the end.

They cheered the winning runner
as he crossed the line first place.
Head high and proud and happy;
no falling; no disgrace.

But when the fallen youngster
crossed the line, last place,
The crowd gave him the greater cheer
for finishing the race!

And even though he came in last,
with head bowed low, unproud;
You would have thought he'd won the race
to listen to the crowd.
And to his dad he sadly said,
"I didn't do so well."
"To me you won," his father said,
"You rose each time you fell."

And when things seem dark and hard
and difficult to face,
The memory of that little boy
helps me with my own race.
For all of life is like that race,
with ups and downs and all,
And all you have to do to win
is rise each time you fall.

"Quit! Give up, you're beaten!"
they may shout in my face.
But another voice within me says,
"GET UP AND WIN THE RACE!"

— Delbert H. Groberg

This poem helped me at my lowest low. It may remind you of another man who fell. He fell three times, as a matter of fact. You see, when Jesus carried our cross to pay the price for our sins, He fell three times. But He got up and He finished. All Heaven and Earth will shout His name one day and I'm glad to be part of His heritage.

Chapter 6

Success Stories

I have seen many miracles, and continue to see them daily, for "with God all things are possible." (Matthew 19:26) I must give all the glory to God for using me as an instrument for healing and transformation. In the Bible it says, "but thou shalt remember the Lord thy God: for it is He that giveth thee power to get wealth, that He may establish His covenant which He sware unto thy fathers, as it is this day." (Deuteronomy 8:18)

I absolutely love going to my office, daily, to practice Quantum Neurology® because I continue to see miracle after miracle. It's inspiring to see people come into the office with little or no movement and incredible amounts of pain and frustration, and then leave my office feeling better and sometimes completely healed.

I love it when underperforming athletes come into my office, and after their visit they go to an event and perform their absolute best. They come back in and show me their trophies and medals. They share their stories with me, of major success in all of their accomplishments, and are truly awe-inspiring. But perhaps the most inspiring are the people who come in paralyzed from a spinal cord or brain injury. Helping them to get well and take their very first steps, after years of being in a wheelchair, is extremely gratifying.

Doctors in all medical professions do their best to help their patients get well. They perform life-sustaining techniques. Western medical doctors do really well with crisis care. Sometimes the true miracles happen after the crisis, well after the patient has left the hospital.

I would love to share a story of a lady who means so much to me. She and her husband have both touched my life.

Karen David's Story

Karen is a sixty-one-year-old woman who was diagnosed with paralysis in her legs and partial paralysis in her arms after being involved in an auto accident. In the accident, she broke the C7 vertebra in her neck. C7 is the lowest vertebra in the cervical spine.

When she first arrived at my office, Karen was in a wheelchair. She could not sit up without support and had to be strapped into the chair. She was so paralyzed that if she just leaned over she couldn't hold herself and she would fall to the floor.

Karen was a referral from one of my past head injury patients who had gotten great results. As I remember the story, this patient had presented his case at a Rotary club meeting and shared about how well he was recovering from his brain injury. Karen's husband, Irving, was at this Rotary club meeting and was blown away by the story. He contacted my office and made an appointment for his wife to come in and see me, for which I am very grateful.

When Karen came to see me, she had a cervical fusion of the C-5 through the C7 vertebra in her neck. What makes this story so special to me is that it had been over twelve years since her accident. She had seen every type of medical doctor, physical therapist—every medical professional imaginable—and they had all but given up on her. Though they did their best to get her to the point she was at when we met, it had been twelve years since she had moved a muscle in her legs, she could barely move her arms, and, as I mentioned at the beginning of the story, she couldn't even sit up on her own.

So when we started to work with her, Karen couldn't move any of the myotomes of her legs. Focusing on certain points and using Quantum Neurology® techniques, the first thing we were able to do was to get her to start to move some of those muscles that had been frozen for over twelve years. It wasn't long before she could do kicking motions with her legs and pull her knees up to her chest without our assistance. This was so exciting and beautiful to witness. She still couldn't sit up in a chair because her core musculature was so weakened from the paralysis that if she just leaned over she would tilt and fall. We had to hold her in place every time that we worked with her.

Eventually, we got Karen to a point where her trunk muscles got strong enough for her to sit up, and we could work on her without holding her up and without her having impact on her chair for support. We were able to move her into an iGallop machine that I have in my office. This machine simulates horseback riding. Now, in order to ride a horse and keep from falling, the back and spine must perform hundreds of thousands of little tiny muscular contractions. Most people are able to do this without being aware that they are doing it or even thinking about it, but when you're paralyzed you can't do any of that.

I will never forget the first time we put Karen on the iGallop machine to see if she would be able to stabilize these muscles while going through motions like galloping and trotting. Bless her heart, she looked at her husband and said, "I want Irving to hold my hand." She had full trust in her husband and knew that if she fell he would catch her.

As we turned on the machine and put Karen through all of the different motions and settings, tears came to our eyes. We wept because she was able to stabilize herself. She started to move her arms and legs with ease and I wondered what the next steps were for her. She had not used the muscles in her legs for so long that the muscles had atrophied, and atrophy was associated with the paralysis from her neck.

I spoke with Karen and her husband and we came to the conclusion that what we needed was a LiteGait® machine (a partial-weight-bearing gait therapy device) which could hold the body up without the strength of muscles, and using this machine she could perform exercise with her legs in a fall-free environment (with no worry that she would fall down). This would be great because I couldn't hold her up and do my work at the same time.

With the help of this machine, it wasn't long before Karen had increased her endurance and the swelling had gone down in her ankles due to the non-contraction of the muscles and the rhythmic contractions of the venous blood being pumped back up into her heart. Ordinarily, paralyzed people in wheelchairs don't have that luxury, but when we started working her out on the LiteGait® machine and she started taking steps, one at a time, we noticed that the ankle swelling was not as bad. This weight bearing exercise also opened the door for improvement from the osteoporosis Karen had developed as a paralysis patient. So we were gaining several different things, at one time, by using this LiteGait® machine.

I am so blessed to see what is happening with Karen now. She is getting strength in her legs to the point that when she contracts her muscles you can feel the muscles go into contraction. She now walks three hundred fifty steps on the LiteGait® machine every time she comes into my office. We put her up on a vibrational board, which vibrates from the bottom of her feet to the top of her head, and she does semi-squats. We lower her down, she's able to push up with her body weight, and she does over a hundred squats each time she comes into the office.

I truly believe that with God's help and keeping her on track, Karen will walk again without support. I am honored and blessed to be working with her. She and her husband have referred so many clients to my office, who have also had great results because of this miracle called Quantum Neurology®.

Roger Sims' Story

Roger is a fifty-year-old man. At the age of twenty-three, he and his wife were in a major automobile accident. They hit a telephone pole and the car flipped over. His wife was killed instantly on impact and Roger had a severe and traumatic brain injury. While Roger was hanging upside down in the car, the electrical wires from the pole they hit ignited the gasoline which had poured out of the car onto the ground. The fire spread to the car and two thirds of Roger's body was burned.

When I first saw Roger, it had been twenty-one years since the accident. He was in a wheelchair and had no function on the left side of his body. He had difficulty understanding what was going on around him and his speech was slurred, so I had a hard time understanding what he was trying to say to me.

Roger had exhausted the traditional medical realm of treatments. He had actively participated in physical therapy and really everything that they had but no matter what the doctors tried, no neurological function in his body had been restored. The traditional medical doctors had all but given up and informed Roger that he would be in this state for the rest of his life.

When he came to see me, we immediately went to work to restore the nervous system on the left side of Roger's body. Complete restoration was our goal. He did not have function of the myotomes connected to the lower extremity or the upper extremity. He could make several movements but they were uncontrollable. His motor skills were highly affected by the accident and he just didn't have any control of movement on the left side of his body.

Each time he came to the office and we worked with the left side of his body, Roger became stronger. As the movement improved, so did his speech. With each visit, I could understand him even better than the one before.

Now, I understand every word Roger says and I could not be happier with the results. He recently expressed that he wants to be the Quantum Neurology® poster child and I've got to tell you, I believe that someday, if not really soon, he will be. He is now walking without any assistance. If I hold his hands—and without the LiteGait® machine—he is able to walk several steps without any help. Due to the severe brain injury that he encountered, he does sometimes still lose his balance. We are working with Quantum Neurology® balancing techniques to get the cranial nerves functioning optimally. Our intention is to restore his ability to equalize the balance he lost due to the car accident.

Currently, Roger is able to walk over eight hundred steps on his own with the LiteGait® machine. The machine aids in balance so that Roger can continue to gain strength. When removed from the LiteGait® machine, Roger is able to walk heel-to-toe without falling over.

If you'd like to help him fulfill his desire to be the Quantum Neurology® poster child, you can search for Roger Sims online at www.youtube.com and you will find a video of him walking. This video has thousands of views and Roger often shares that no previous medical treatment or therapy ever helped him like Quantum Neurology® did. With power and determination, he has come a long way in what seems like a short amount of time and I truly believe that we'll have him back to a hundred percent really soon.

There's one thing that I find particularly interesting about Roger's case. At the time of the injury, the surgeons did a tendon transfer on one of his legs. They needed the tendon to assist them in other repairs in his body. When he came to see me and I told him I'd like him to do a toe raise (stand on his toes to lift his body up), he said, "I won't be able to do that."

"Why not?" I asked.

"They did a tendon transfer on my Achilles tendon and I don't think I can do that."

I chuckled, looked at him, and said, "Roger, just do it!"

He now does a hundred toe raises every time he visits my office and the tendon in that leg has been fully restored. Quite simply, it grew back. This is a miracle in itself.

Roger is now able to function at a much higher capacity. He talks well, he functions well, he has restored lost motor skills, and he is just rocking and rolling. I believe he will be the first person I've ever seen go from paralysis in a wheelchair to walking on his own, over twenty years after a tragic accident. Typically, physical damage is permanent if it has been longer than two years from the time a trauma occurred. That's what the medical doctors tell the patients.

When I use Quantum Neurology® techniques with my patients, I always give them something to build on. I can remember a time in the past when Roger was getting discouraged. He felt the results were coming too slowly and so I read him the poem, "The Race," which I shared with you in Chapter 5. It encouraged him to soldier on and his attitude instantly changed back to being positive. Roger is a fighter by nature and I truly believe that both he and Karen David will walk at a hundred percent on their own someday. I want to give God all the praise and glory for that.

Dr. Sue Lein's Story

Dr. Sue Lein is sixty-seven years old and is an incredible person.

Like Karen David, she was also referred to my office by Irving David. Irving has referred many patients to our office because he's so excited and happy to share his wife's miracle with everyone he meets. Due to Irving's efforts, I have not advertised my business in over ten years. I'm grateful for Irving and I'm so glad that he sent Dr. Sue to our office.

Seventeen years before I met her, Dr. Sue had been diagnosed with MSA (Multiple Systems Atrophy). Since MSA is a disease which often results from having had encephalitis, Dr. Sue determined that while she was training for a marathon she had been bitten by a mosquito which was carrying the encephalitis germ. She was diagnosed with the St. Louis variety of encephalitis, which is the worst you can get. The average lifespan, after contracting St. Louis encephalitis, is two years.

At the time of her diagnosis, Dr. Sue was cared for by a medical doctor at an MSA center. Ten years later (seven years before we met), she made the life-saving decision to see Dr. Robert Martinez, a neurologist, who prescribed the muscle relaxer, baclofen. His idea of relaxing her muscles ended up being exactly what her body needed for her to survive the life span estimate from the medical doctors.

One of my chiropractic assistants, Sandra Menard, worked as a nurse for a medical doctor for twelve years and has been with me for over eight. Sandra is one of the most positive people I know. She knows and believes that everyone can get well. The only time I heard her say anything negative was when she first met Dr. Sue. Sandra came down the hall, looked at me, and said, "Doc, I don't think you're going to be able to help this one."

"Let's just see what happens," I replied.

When I first saw Sue Lein, she was bent at the waist by ninety degrees and her head was just a little bit above her knees. She had been stuck in that position for over seventeen years. She had no pain. As a matter of fact, she couldn't feel anything at all. I guess it was partly due to the baclofen drug, which had led them to install a pump in her body to give her this medicine consistently. This had probably saved her life in the beginning, but over time her quality of life was becoming less and less. She was frozen in this bent position and couldn't do anything.

After examining Sue Lein and using Quantum Neurology® techniques, I was able to find the weaknesses in her nervous system. I looked at Sue and I told her, "I have to warn you about something. Once we turn these nerves back on, the first thing that may come back is pain."

"Oh, I wish that I had pain. You don't understand…I can't feel anything."

"Be careful what you wish for because you may just get it," I said as we continued to work on her and set her up a second appointment.

When she returned for her second appointment, she looked at me and said, "Turn the pain off. Turn the pain off."

"I told you that once you turn nerves back on, the first thing that returns is the pain."

But pain is not a bad thing, believe it or not. It's actually the body's response to it coming back to life. Have you ever slept on your arm long enough to cut off the blood flow (nerve supply) to that arm? You wake up and you can't feel your arm because it's numb, right? You shake it and shake it and sooner or later it starts circulating the nerves to come back, and sometimes when that happens it's a little painful getting back to normal. This is what happened with Dr. Sue. Over seventeen years of not feeling anything and then, suddenly, we turned the nerves back on, which caused her to feel some serious pain.

I couldn't figure out how she could be in so much pain and still be smiling. She looked at me and said, "Look at this." She was sitting up straight, had lifted her head up, and was looking straight at the ceiling. "I haven't been able to do that for seventeen years, Dr. Chauvin."

I thought to myself, *wow, that's so cool!*

The more we worked with Dr. Sue, the more she improved. Her posture improved and people started saying things like, "I didn't know you were that tall, Sue." Not only did these results improve her overall appearance, but her legs started getting stronger and stronger.

Remember that before she was diagnosed with MSA, she was a marathon runner. This is a woman who was used to exercising daily and all of a sudden she couldn't sit up straight. She was glad to be on the mend and willing to do what was necessary to get back to perfect health. The doctors had given her just two years to live and now, seventeen years later, God has given her life back to her. People have asked her, "Did you get a face lift? You look so much younger."

She shared this with me, laughing. "Can you believe that they thought I had a face lift?" This is not surprising to me because she does look twenty-five years younger than the first time I saw her.

Quantum Neurology® is a nerve rehabilitation technique that works. It's so powerful. I've seen many people get up from their wheelchairs and walk. And I've seen many people, like Dr. Sue, get their lives back. She no longer has the baclofen pump—she no longer takes any baclofen—and her medical doctors have told her that she no longer has MSA. As far as I know, she's the only person who has ever lived to tell that story. MSA is said to not go away…ever. One is not supposed to live at all, let alone live a life of quality and good health.

One day, Dr. Sue came into my office with a piece of paper in her hand. "Edward, look at this." She waved the paper around. "My doctor just did this blood test and he tells me that I don't have leukemia anymore."

"Wow! You mean God could have used me for a miracle such as this?" I looked at the paper and, sure enough, the blood test confirmed that she no longer had leukemia. Now I'm not trying to say that we're going to treat all leukemia patients or that Quantum Neurology® is the answer to it, but in Sue Lein's case, it happened.

In working with Sue, I used a very unique Quantum Neurology® technique, developed by Dr. George Gonzalez, called "holographic transfer," in which we treated her DNA with her son's DNA. When I explained to her that her son had the same DNA and we could use it, she said, "My son is healthy and I'm sure he'll do it, but he lives in Minnesota."

I told Sue to have her son take skin scrapings from the inside of his mouth with cotton swabs, put the cotton swabs in a zippered plastic bag, and send them to us. When the samples arrived, I took her son's DNA and used it to treat her DNA. Two weeks later, her blood values went back to normal.

This technique stretched me beyond my training. It far surpasses what people think a chiropractor can do. I'm not trying to say that chiropractic cures all diseases, but I am saying that Quantum Neurology® was the force inside of Sue that caused her body to go back to normal. She exercises four to five times a week now. She's looking better, feeling better, and comes back every couple of weeks with another story of improvement.

I could go on and on sharing the miracles I've seen in my office, thanks to God and Quantum Neurology®. Witnessing miracles, on a daily basis, makes my life very rewarding. I am so amazed by Dr. Sue's story and so many others I am able to tell. I've seen blind people get their sight back…people talking who couldn't speak…paralyzed people getting up out of their wheelchairs and walking. The bible says, "and these signs shall follow them that believe; in my name shall they cast out devils; they shall speak with new tongues…they shall lay hands on the sick, and they shall recover." (Mark 16:17-18) I truly believe that God is using Quantum Neurology® and Quantum Neurology® practitioners to achieve this. We just need to give God all the glory and keep pursuing these techniques that are helping sick people to get well.

Chapter 7

Quantum Neurology®
and the Future of
Chiropractic Care

I have practiced chiropractic for thirty years now and I love this great profession. In a little over a hundred years, chiropractic has proven itself to be the number one treatment for lower back and neck related problems, without the use of drugs or surgery. I have seen a lot of change in thirty years.

When I first got out of chiropractic college in 1981, people were scared to come into a chiropractor's office. Medical doctors would not refer patients to us at all and when we needed an MRI or a CT scan to rule out other pathologies than just spinal misalignments causing nerve pinching, it was hard to get the hospitals to run those tests.

Today this has changed because chiropractic has produced some very impressive results. It has proven to stand the test of time. Quantum Neurology® chiropractic has just started to produce case studies that are nothing less than miracles. We don't know what to call them because with standard treatments the medical and chiropractic fields have never seen these types of miracles before.

I was introduced to Dr. George Gonzalez in 2002 at a seminar in Dallas, Texas and I thank God for him every day. His method of evaluating the nervous system using Quantum Neurology®, and applying chiropractic treatments with light therapy, will be the beginning of a new form of healing that will affect the whole world. I see that someday in the near future, medical doctors, chiropractors, and all health care practitioners will have to have some degree of knowledge of Quantum Neurology® so they can evaluate the nervous system to discover the problems that need to be treated.

When I was at the seminar in Dallas, I had no idea that I would be forever changed by my attendance. Upon leaving the event, I was better at applying chiropractic principles and the adjustments that I gave became more specific, with a greater, and measurable, response. I was able to show the patients instant results that reached far beyond the popping noise that comes from the typical chiropractic adjustment to relieve the nerve interference.

We used to show our patients "before" and "after" x-rays with visible changes that could be measured, but it took some three to six months of care to show them those results. I'm not saying there isn't value in the chiropractic adjustment itself; I thank God for that because it helps so many people. But in the three to six months that I was treating my patients, they would be worrying themselves sick. They'd constantly be asking me fear based questions, expecting to hear answers that would calm them down.

Once I started using the Quantum Neurology® techniques, I was able to show my patients results not only instantly, but consistently, until the patients came into full recovery. I am so thankful for Quantum Neurology® because I get to show them on the first treatment that they're making progress. I truly believe that Quantum Neurology® should be taught in every chiropractic college so that people will have less nerve interference and chiropractic will make another quantum leap into the future.

Quantum Neurology® can easily help some of the physical problems that I would never have attempted to treat using strictly chiropractic adjustments. One example is cranial nerve deficits. I remember studying cranial nerves in chiropractic college. We learned to evaluate patients to see if they could perform these cranial nerve responses and if they couldn't, there was no adjustment for that. We just referred them out for testing to make sure we ruled out brain injuries, strokes, tumors, and anything else that was nervous system related. Cranial nerve deficits show up in many people, with little hope that conventional medicine, or chiropractic, can help. Some that are very familiar to my office are Bell's palsy (a paralysis on the side of the face), attention deficit disorder (ADD), attention deficit hyperactive disorder (ADHD), temporomandibular joint disorder (TMJD), and autism. Sometimes these syndromes are alleviated quickly, using Quantum Neurology®, by evaluation and treatment of these particular cranial nerves. I have seen instant improvement in eyesight and in some cases hearing losses have been restored. Swallowing is a function we rarely think about but is incredibly important. I have seen patients who had surgery, lost their ability to swallow, and, using Quantum Neurology® techniques, were able to fully regain their swallowing function.

We also use Quantum Neurology® techniques to treat allergies. There are many cases in which patients come into the office looking for relief from food allergies. In my office, we've treated allergies to eggs, milk, and many other foods. Before treatment, if they ate the foods they were allergic to these patients would have a neurological response. Once treated, they were able to eat the same foods with no negative neurological responses. I've seen a few food allergy cases in which these treatments have actually saved a patient's life. Airborne allergies are common in South Louisiana and Quantum Neurology® allows these patients to be desensitized to these allergens quickly and effectively, without drugs, needles, or surgery. After treatment, they are able to lead a normal, allergy-free life.

Another common ailment we treat in our office is shingles, which is a viral infection in the nerve root and shows up as a very painful skin rash. Shingles usually appears in a band, a strip, or a small area on one side of the face or in the rib cage area. Usually, the rash breaks out with pustules and, using Quantum Neurology® techniques, we are able to take some of the serum from one of the pustules and treat it as an allergen. Most of the time, after completion of the treatment, the pain subsides and the patient is completely healed within a few days to a few weeks.

Another Quantum Neurology® technique I use in my practice is holographic transfer. In Chapter 6, I told you about Sue Lein, one of my miracle patients. Sue had multiple systems atrophy and leukemia for many years before coming to see me. Her son was a very healthy young man, so we took a sample of his DNA (by swabbing the inside of his mouth) and shipped it from where he was in Minnesota down to my office in Louisiana. Because his DNA and her DNA were genetically matched, we were able to activate recognition with her nervous system. Within two weeks, her blood chemistry went to normal standards. She has made a remarkable recovery, thanks to this incredible holographic transfer technique. I see this technique being used in the future to handle all types of blood-borne pathologies, and others for which we have no treatment at this point.

I've seen other Quantum Neurology® doctors breaking ground with their techniques as well. Two doctors who have been doing great work are James Sheen from Nebraska and Dr. Chris Cormier, a friend of mine from Lafayette, Louisiana. They are both working with the periodic table of elements and getting extraordinary results with allergies and autoimmune disorders related to particular elements. Going forth into the future, I see that as being something very big…that we will be able to treat all types of incurable, and chronic, disorders, with great results.

Another technique that shows promise is a fungus protocol I've been working on. I had a dream and in that dream, I talked to God. He told me that leprosy was caused by a fungus which kills the nerve endings in the hands and feet, and that this is why you see people with leprosy in the movies, or in real life, who have lost fingers, toes, or even their nose. For years, many doctors have believed that it was bacterial, so they have treated it with antibiotics and it has gone away. But in this dream, God told me that all neuropathies are caused by funguses. This got me interested enough to start fooling around with it myself and I have come to find out that it was the truth.

When Sue Lein presented with numbness in her feet, which she'd had for eighteen years before coming to my office, she couldn't feel them at all. We were able to bring back neurological function to every part of her body except her feet. You could stick a pin in her feet and she still couldn't feel them, so I developed this fungus protocol for her.

Sue had been treated with antibiotics over and over again. At some point, maybe she was treated with antibiotics for a bacterial infection and she got well and her body said, *oh, this is good…*her nervous system decided, *this antibiotic is good for me*, so it held onto it until it became an addiction. The body didn't want to get rid of it, it just wanted to keep holding onto it. Maybe this type of antibiotic was a fungus and actually caused a disconnection between Sue's nervous system and her feet so that she couldn't feel anything.

So here's what we did: I took a culture of Sue's saliva, early in the morning, using cotton balls, sugar, and water and kept it in the darkness. Within seven to ten days, this fungus was growing inside the bag. It was black and almost coming outside of the bag. As a matter fact, my chiropractic assistant, Sandra, said, "Oh, Doc, I'm afraid to touch that thing." It was really bad.

Next, we treated Sue with this fungus protocol for her feet. She started getting sensation back into her feet right away and within a few weeks she had regained full function back to her feet. She shared things like, "My God! I can feel my feet again. I can go upstairs. I can feel everything in my feet." We were all really excited.

A few weeks later, Sue got a bacterial infection, went to see her M.D., and, of course, he treated her with another round of antibiotics. The interesting thing about this was that after she was treated with antibiotics, all the numbness came back to her feet. The neuropathy was back, so we treated her, again, with this fungus protocol that we had developed and she got back the feeling in her feet again.

I believe that in the future, all neuropathy patients, including diabetic neuropathies and MSA patients like Sue, will be able to be helped using this fungus protocol. We have had success but there is still much to be done. Just to be clear, this is chiropractic using light therapy. It is not that we are treating infections, because chiropractors don't treat infections in the state of Louisiana. But in a neurological sense, we helped the neuropathy and brought back neurological functions in Sue's feet, so it still is within the scope of our practice.

In the future, I see hospitals with medical doctors and chiropractors working together, both being trained in Quantum Neurology® to enhance the body's recuperative ability to heal itself, instead of using drugs, surgery, or chiropractic adjustment for everything. A better evaluation and a better treatment will be made available to help people get well. This is how I see the future of chiropractic and Quantum Neurology®.

Conclusion

It is my hope that after reading this book, you will quit worrying yourself sick about your health and you will realize that you need to make a change for the better in your life.

This book is filled with tips to make it easy but rest assured, "with God all things are possible." (Matthew 19:26) No matter where you are in the process—whether you're already healthy or you're seeking to gain your health back—you can start, from this point forward, to direct your own path back to health, back to God, and into a bright future.

I pray, in the name of Jesus, that you will take this message and bring it out with you to affect other people…not just for yourself but for your family, your friends, and whomever you can think of. You can even affect your enemies by giving them something positive so they can be healthy…or maybe not hate you…or maybe even make friends with you. And maybe by doing this, you can be all that God wants you to be.

Thank you!

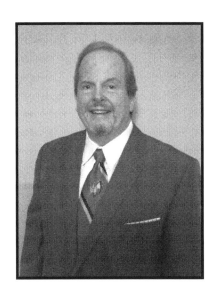

About the Author

Edward Chauvin, D.C., graduated with honors (cum laude) from Palmer Chiropractic College in 1981. He has practiced chiropractic for thirty years. He is a native of Louisiana and the first chiropractor in his family.

In 2002, Dr. Chauvin met Dr. George Gonzalez and continued to study Quantum Neurology® to become the seventh Quantum Neurologist™ in the world. He was also honored by Dr. Gonzalez for being part of an FDA study on the GRT lite being approved to treat carpal tunnel, and shoulder and neck problems. He has helped thousands of patients over the years, using chiropractic techniques, and has wonderful success with many of the neurological disorders that are not typically thought to be helped by chiropractic adjustments.

Dr. Chauvin is a member of the American Chiropractic Association and the Chiropractic Association of Louisiana. He has been honored in the past with the Obelisk Award, by Kats Management Services, for educating patients to the benefits of chiropractic care. He has received awards in Quantum Neurology® for case studies on brain and spinal cord injuries, and for his work with neurotoxic fungus.

Dr. Chauvin's office is located at:

1000 Wildcat Drive
Abbeville, Louisiana 70510
Phone: (337) 893-5252